Extreme Dreaming

EXTREME DREAMING

Decode Your Nightmares and Awaken Your Wisdom Within

Theresa Cheung

GODSFIELD

First published in Great Britain in 2026 by Godsfield Press, an imprint of
Octopus Publishing Group Ltd
Carmelite House
50 Victoria Embankment
London EC4Y 0DZ
www.octopusbooks.co.uk

An Hachette UK Company
www.hachette.co.uk

The authorized representative in the EEA is Hachette Ireland,
8 Castlecourt Centre, Dublin 15, D15 XTP3, Ireland (email: info@hbgi.ie)

Distributed in the US by Hachette Book Group
1290 Avenue of the Americas, 4th and 5th Floors
New York, NY 10104

Distributed in Canada by Canadian Manda Group
664 Annette St., Toronto, Ontario, Canada M6S 2C8

ISBN: 978-1-84181-616-6
eISBN: 978-1-84181-617-3

A CIP catalogue record for this book is available from the British Library.

Typeset in 11.75/18pt Heldane Text by Six Red Marbles UK, Thetford, Norfolk

Printed and bound in Great Britain.

1 3 5 7 9 10 8 6 4 2

Commissioning Editor: Louisa Johnson
Project Editor: Rimsha Falak
Copy Editor: Monica Hope
Art Director: Yasia Williams
Production Managers: Lucy Carter & Nic Jones

This FSC® label means that materials used for the
product have been responsibly sourced.

MIX
Paper | Supporting responsible forestry
FSC® C104740

For the spirit of Mary Shelley (1797–1851), author of Frankenstein, whose 'undying' creation grew from a waking nightmare and showed that even the most unsettling dreams and visions can be transformed into enduring acts of imagination and creation.

Contents

Introduction

YOUR WORST NIGHTMARE

What's your worst nightmare?

The kind that hurls you awake in the dead of the night, heart pounding, drenched in sweat and convinced, for a few seconds, that your life is over or your mind has snapped because it felt so real? The kind that you can recall in vivid detail days, months or even years afterwards.

Maybe your worst nightmare is waking in the early hours of the morning, fists clenched tight, utterly convinced a loved one has died. You saw it clearly in your dream: a violent car crash, shattering glass, twisted metal and their lifeless body lying just beyond reach. You sit frozen, caught between the terrifying images conjured up by your mind and the desperate hope it was only a nightmare. Was the crushing weight of dread and fear for a loved one's safety that lingers long after you've opened your eyes, blurring the lines between dream and reality, some kind of warning?

Or imagine this: the sharp, scraping sound of shattering glass in your bedroom, followed by a cold rush of breath as a monstrous spider, bigger than any you've ever seen before, crashes through your window. Its bloodshot eyes gleam with malevolent intent and long, writhing tentacles slither towards you from its grotesque body, reaching, grasping. On waking, you lie paralysed in a cold sweat, unable to move, the fear so visceral it feels like it might eat you from the inside out. Only after several trembling moments do you convince yourself it's just a nightmare – but the terror clings like a shadow.

Have you ever been trapped in a nightmare where you're suddenly naked in a crowded place, exposed and vulnerable, everyone's judgemental eyes burning into you? Or buried alive, suffocating beneath the cold, unyielding earth, panic clawing at your throat? Or frozen in a silent scream, trying to get someone – anyone – to hear or notice you but to no avail? Maybe you are desperately chased by faceless strangers or savage wild animals that are always closing in, no matter how fast you run. Or perhaps you're haunted by the twisted and all-too-common dream scenario of burying a dead body and then waking up unable to remember where you hid it, a gnawing fear that it's still out there, buried in the dark but soon to be exposed.

What about being trapped inside your own burning home? The flames licking closer, the smoke filling your lungs, while from somewhere inside you hear a terrified baby scream and your feet feel rooted to the spot, like they're encased in concrete, helpless to save the helpless. Or do you see blood everywhere and it takes you a while to realize it is *you* who has been wounded or shot? Perhaps you are in a tiny, windowless prison cell and being asked for your 'last meal' request before your execution by a firing squad; or maybe you find yourself inexplicably surrounded by severed body parts, some of which belong to you.

Have you ever dreamed of betrayal so raw it shakes you awake? Watching in slow motion as your partner cheats on you with someone you know and trust, the image burning into your mind. Or losing your children in a chaotic, bustling shopping centre, every face a stranger's, every turn leading to a dead end. Or sinking, slowly and silently, beneath dark water that swallows all sound and drags you mercilessly to the depths. Maybe you're trapped in mud or quicksand, sinking deeper, or being ripped apart by wild beasts, your cries swallowed by the dense forest. Or you are back in school, the torment of bullying replaying endlessly. Perhaps you struggle to perform the most basic tasks, like opening your locker, and everyone is laughing at your incompetence. Then your hair starts to fall out in clumps, your face melts or your teeth are crumbling and falling out one by one – each loss another small horror.

Maybe your worst nightmare is snakes coiling and hissing all around, their cold bodies pressing in with no escape? Or those scary clowns, their painted faces twisted into grotesque smiles as they taunt you with cruel laughter. Or you're caught in the crushing force of a tsunami and swept away to certain death, or falling headfirst from a dizzying height, the ground rushing up to meet you. Maybe there are crawling bugs – thousands of them – covering your skin, burrowing into your flesh. Perhaps dead birds or stones are raining down on you from the sky, or you find yourself facing apocalypse, utterly alone on a barren Earth, the last living soul wandering through endless dead bodies and ruins.

Any of these scenarios resonate? Even if you can't recall dreaming them as described, did they send a shiver of inexplicable recognition down your spine?

Nightmares have long held a haunting power over us. They don't just frighten – they reveal, disturb and sometimes even inspire us. *Frankenstein*, perhaps the most enduring horror story ever written, was born from a nightmare the author Mary Shelley had on a storm-swept night – a timeless night vision that refuses to die. The story follows a young, ambitious scientist who creates life from dead matter, only to be horrified by the unnatural creature he has unleashed. That same lingering feeling of impending darkness, and the disturbing, distorted spark of something unnatural coming alive in the shadows, pulses through the night visions that people repeatedly share with me.

Chances are at least one of those nightmare scenarios did strike a chord with you. That's because they are among the most common nightmare scenarios or stories reported to dream researchers like me. I've been sent thousands of night horrors over the years – petrifying fragments of the subconscious from people all over the world. My inbox continually overflows with whispered secrets, midnight monsters and other dark echoes that emerge only in the twisted world of the nightmare. From these accounts, I've built a vast, ever-expanding archive – a kind of nightfright database or grisly library of horrors that is filled with some of the most chilling dream terrors imaginable. Although every nightmare sent to me is utterly unique, many have familiar themes that strangely repeat.

Even if you haven't (yet) personally dreamed any of these scenarios, you will still recognize the feeling of terror running through them, perhaps the same terror that fuels your own waking fears. The more bizarre your dream, the more it hints at deep fears and unresolved conflicts lurking in your subconscious. But nightmares are more than just bizarre. They are psychologically scarring and often deeply unsettling; grotesque images and stories designed to imprison your thoughts long after dawn breaks.

Nightmares do feel like a savage warning to the dreamer – a symbolic maiming or message from the dark depths of the unconscious that should not be ignored. We don't always fully understand them, but one thing is certain: the brutal symbolism of the dream wakes us the hell up. And it keeps us awake, fearful of its return. The memory of it may still be burned in our minds years later, recalled more vividly than anything happening in our waking life at the time.

What's even more unnerving is that nightmares don't happen only while you are sleeping. Sometimes, they can spill over into your waking moments when intrusive and unwanted thoughts strike unawares. Have you ever experienced that sudden, irrational urge to leap from a great height, even while knowing, rationally, that you would never act on it? That fleeting 'death wish' impulse to fall, to plunge into darkness, gives us a chilling glimpse into how our minds can suddenly and inexplicably leap into unfathomable realms beyond our conscious control. It's a stark reminder that the boundary between dreams and reality is thinner than we think. The shadows hiding in our minds always seem to be biding their time, waiting behind the scenes for an opportunity to pounce.

Nightmares Need a PR Team

Over the many decades I've spent writing and teaching about dream healing, I've received countless messages from people – desperate, disturbed and sometimes quietly ashamed – all asking the same question: 'What on earth does this nightmare mean?' They've scoured books, websites and forums in search of clarity, only to find themselves empty-handed. Often, they're met with platitudes about dream positivity, simplistic wish-fulfilment theories or symbolism so vague it slips through their fingers like fine sand.

That's why this book exists: to bring clarity to the murky realm of nightmares – why we have them, what they're truly saying and how they can become powerful tools for inner healing.

The inspiration for this book came, fittingly, in the dead of night. I awoke with a start consumed with the memory of a dark dream in which I walked a long corridor lined with mirrors. None of them reflected me. Instead, each showed a different face – some weeping, some screaming, some melting, some skeletal, some frozen – all of them inexplicably filled with dread. I felt watched by a hundred versions of sorrow and fear. When I tried to run, the corridor folded inwards like a maze with no exit. Just before waking, the last mirror cracked and a voice whispered: *You can't outrun your dreams.*

That nightmare shook me, not just because of its terror but because of the instant 'aha' moment of recognition it brought. Every day, people send me their dreams, hoping for understanding, and I do my best to respond with dream-decoding advice. What I hadn't fully grasped until that moment was just how many of those dreams are dark, nightmarish and charged with raw emotional pain: being chased, lost, falling, dying or battling dark and threatening forces. For years, I'd been guiding others towards the healing power of their dreams, but I hadn't truly asked myself: why are so many of us dreaming so darkly and what are our collective nightmares really trying to say?

Those questions held me long after dawn. In the days that followed, I began revisiting my own dream journals and the database of dreams others had shared with me. Very soon, a pattern emerged – one I'd previously overlooked or hadn't wanted to acknowledge. These weren't just strange stories. They were pain wrapped in symbolism, trauma hidden in metaphor, fear begging to be seen, heard and understood. In another sudden moment of clarity, everything aligned: bad dreams don't come to hurt or haunt us – they arrive at exactly the right time and with a clear mission. They show up when we're ready for their honesty and when a window for transformation is opening in our waking lives.

That's when I realized: nightmares need some serious PR. There's no such thing as a terrifying dream; there is only a terrified dreamer. Nightmares are like a brutally honest friend who during times of uncertainty will tell you what you *need* to hear, not what you *want* to hear. Nightmares are your honest reality check, an inner emergency-broadcast system, sounding the alarm when it matters most, while you still have a chance to understand their truth and take the best course of action. I like to think of nightmares as just 'extreme dreams'; hence the title of this book.

In that sense, extreme dreams are both a wakeup call and a signal that you're closer to healing than you might think. If you can find the courage to face and work with them, real transformation and personal power lie ahead. If you ignore them, the denial and delusion continue and, if left unaddressed, may carry you into dangerous territory. So, if you take just one thing away, let it be this: a nightmare is not a bad omen. It could represent the most important and even the most auspicious shift in your inner life. A chance to evolve, to become a more self-aware and wiser version of yourself.

Sweet Dreams or Beautiful Nightmares?

We're taught to wish each other 'sweet dreams' before bed, as though sleep should bring only peace and beauty. But sweet dreams are rare. Nighttime isn't a static period of blissful rest – it's a time of mental motion. Research shows that most of our dreams are anxiety-laden, filled with fear and distress; if they're not full-blown nightmares, then they're teetering on the edge of becoming them. The comforting 'sweet dreams' we wish one another are the exception. Bad dreams, it seems, are the norm. For most of us, the night is a battleground where our deepest fears repeatedly play out behind our eyes in vivid, extreme detail. We carry vast, unresolved emotional worlds into sleep. What emerges, especially in disturbing dreams, reveals what our waking selves have pushed aside but that must surface for healing to begin.

This book is not about avoiding those unsettling dreams; it's about facing and understanding their message. It's both your guide and companion through the night. My aim isn't to eliminate distressing dreams – I would not 'dream' of doing that, because the opportunity for personal growth they offer is far too valuable. Instead, I want to help you navigate them, so that what once terrified you begins to heal and even empower you.

It's time to stop turning away from the shadows in our dreaming minds. It's time to stop fearing the dark. This is your precious opportunity to explore the nightmares we try to forget, the dreams we're afraid to name and the deeper truths buried within them. My goal is not only to illuminate the hidden meanings of your nightmares but also to give you practical tools to work with them, transform them and reclaim the surprising wisdom they carry.

Bad Dreams Linger

The sting of bad dreams lingers. We carry their emotional aftershock into our waking lives, feeling shaken, unsettled or ashamed. Their content often clashes with our self-image. Who wants to admit dreaming of monstrosities, betrayal or madness? Who wants to confront a version of themselves that is lost, broken or consumed by rage? So, we suppress them. We dismiss them. We hope they vanish.

But they don't. Not really. Because the dreaming mind isn't concerned with comfort – it's concerned with truth. It seeks to awaken, to challenge, to jolt us into greater self-awareness. And the hard truth is this: running from nightmares only strengthens their grip. You must face them – eyes wide shut and eye wide open. Listen to them. Let them speak their clear and present truth to you. You can't release and move forward from them unless you first understand their message.

This is the brave heart of the book you now hold: even the most grotesque, spine-chilling dreams aren't here to hurt you. They're here to help you heal. They are messages from your innermost self, urgent cries for attention, asking to be acknowledged, integrated and transformed. Often, gentler dreams have come before them, bearing similar wisdom – but we have forgotten them, dismissed them or failed to reflect. So, the dreams have no choice but to become extreme and grow louder, more vivid, more intense.

When you dare to engage with your nightmares, they can lead you to powerful emotional insight, deep personal growth and even spiritual awakening. They ask you to face the fears you've buried, the truths you've avoided, the pain you've tried to outrun. And when you do, something astonishing can happen: the monster may become a protector. The haunted house a sanctuary. The darkness a source of unexpected light.

This book is your invitation to journey into your own heart of darkness – not to suffer, but to understand and heal. Not to fear, but to transform. Because hidden within your most disturbing dreams is a breathtaking secret: they are not just stories of horror. In their darkness, an unexpected guide appears. Someone who knows the way. That's what your bad dreams can become: your wisest mentors, fiercest protectors and truest allies. They shine their eerie light when you most need it. And here lies the paradox: the darker the dream, the deeper the wisdom and the greater its power to trigger self-reflection and lead you towards the light. Shine on.

Blind trust: a dream-analysis example

The 'blind trust' nightmare scenario described below is based on numerous accounts that have been submitted to me by different dreamers, each unaware of the others. The details vary slightly – sometimes the dream involves limbs rather than the eyes – but the core dream theme remains the same. That's what makes this night vision so arresting: it isn't just one person's private hell. It's a recurring echo, a collective scream from the darkness. If you had a nightmare with a similar storyline, would it become your worst one too?

Let this dream analysis serve as an example: by the end of this book, you will be able to decode such scream-inducing dreams with the same level of clarity and insight. More than that, you will be able to approach a dream like this with curiosity rather than fear.

Remind yourself that what unfolds here isn't real. It didn't happen. It is just a very, very bad dream . . .

It always starts the same way: the dreamer realizes they've lost vision in one eye. It's not painful, just gone. A dark void. Covered by a patch. Useless. Then, a doctor or surgeon appears, faceless, emotionless, with his head wrapped tightly in a thin, stocking-like mask that blurs all his features. He tells the dreamer that their visionless eye is fatally infected. It must be removed immediately, or they will die. There's no resistance from the dreamer. After all, the surgeon is an expert in these things and what's the point of keeping a dead eye?

Suddenly, they're in a hospital, under cold fluorescent lights. The operating room hums and stutters like a machine on the edge of malfunction. Just before the dreamer goes under, panic takes hold. The masked surgeon is leaning over them with a scalpel.

'It's this eye,' the dreamer pleads, clutching the surgeon's arm and pointing at the sightless eye. 'Please, take this one. Not the other one.'

The surgeon's voice is flat, impassive.

'Yes, of course. Why would we remove a healthy eye?'

Then blackness.

When the dreamer awakes, their head is cocooned in bandages. Silence stretches. Nothingness. No pain. No feeling. No vision. No colour. Just dark.

The masked doctor returns and begins unwrapping the gauze with slow, deliberate fingers. Then he pauses.

'The operation was a success. Tell me what you can see,' he says.

'I don't know,' the dreamer replies, heart thudding. 'There's still more bandage you need to remove . . . I can't see anything yet.'

But the doctor doesn't speak.

Fear spikes. The dreamer tears at their face, desperate to rip off the remaining wrappings, only to discover that there are none left. The bandages are gone. So is the light.

The wrong eye has been taken. Now, total darkness. Blindness.

Panic blooms into full hysteria. The scream that follows cracks through the fabric of the dream, jolting the dreamer wide awake in a pitch-black room. Still living in the grip of their nightmare, they scramble for the light, clawing at the switch. When it flickers on, they rush to a mirror and only then, staring into their reflection, do they confirm the truth: both eyes are still there. Everything is fine. It was a very bad dream.

But the memory of the night horror doesn't fade for the dreamer. They stand there for quite a while, hands trembling, their heart pounding as if it knows something alarming that they don't.

Why is this recurring nightmare scenario so deeply disorienting?

Because at its core, it's not just about the fear of blindness or an operation going spectacularly wrong – it's about the deeper terror of betrayal by someone we automatically trust. The doctor/surgeon, a symbol of healing and authority, becomes the agent of irreversible harm. There is no overt violence, no struggle. Only the quiet horror of submission, of agreeing to something because a trusted source said it was necessary. This is a nightmare about the perils and vulnerability of literal and symbolic blind trust. Trust in a figure who offers safety, speaks with calm assurance and then quietly leads you into darkness.

And once that unquestioning trust is broken in the world of the dream, the fear lingers. Because who can you trust, if not those who are meant to protect you? The psychological wound runs deep, touching on childhood fears of helplessness, adult fears of misjudgement and a universal dread that one day you might unsuspectingly give away your trust – and therefore your power – to someone who doesn't deserve it, realizing the cost only when it's far too late to recover what has been lost.

How to Read This Book

With courage. But also with care.

Nightmare content can be intense and may stir up strong emotions. I am a dream expert, but I am not a mental-health professional – so if at any point you find yourself feeling overwhelmed, please pause, take a breath and reach out to a trusted friend, therapist, counsellor or your GP. You don't have to do this work alone.

That said, I encourage you to read this book all the way through the first time, letting the shocking stories, surprising tools and sensational insights wash all over you. Then return to the beginning and read it again but this time mindfully, fully engaging with all the self-help practices and dreamwork techniques in each chapter. Make this more than a book. Make it your heroic journey, your victory over darkness.

What Lies Ahead

In the coming chapters, you'll be taken deep into the heart of the tormented world of your worst nightmares – what they are, why we have them and how they can become surprising sources of insight, healing and creativity.

Chapter One begins with the science and psychology behind extreme dreams and explores how nightmares differ from ordinary dreams and night terrors. You'll discover how working with bad dreams can support your emotional wellbeing. Practical tools like journalling and drawing will help you begin working with your bad dreams directly.

Chapter Two will unpack the secret meanings of nightmares through a simple yet powerful seven-step method of interpretation you can apply to every bad (and good) dream. You'll learn to trace their messages back to your waking life. Through reflection, free association and guided questions, you'll uncover the hidden wisdom buried in even the most distressing dreams.

From there, Chapter Three leaps into the shadow self – those disowned parts of you that love to play the leading roles in nightmares. You'll meet your inner child, dive headfirst into the notion of projection and begin transforming fear into self-awareness. This chapter also explores shadow or intrusive thoughts that can inexplicably break through when you are awake; it discusses what these thoughts mean and what you can do to ease them when they strike.

In Chapter Four, you'll investigate the wild and wonderful potential of liminal states for your personal growth and how to incubate and reprogramme your dreams to help you find meaning and healing. Death as a long-running theme in dreams is the super-intense and often reported nightmare theme of Chapter Five. Chapter Six looks to the future: helping children cope with 'bad' dreams, understanding how nightmares change across the lifespan, how fears can manifest both nightmares and a happier life and, last but not least, how to recognize the hallmarks of so-called 'psychic' dreams – afterlife, telepathic and precognitive night visions.

Finally, the dark terrain of recurring extreme-dream themes will be decoded in Chapter Seven, in an easy-to-reference A–Z of the 101 nightmare scenarios that are most commonly reported to dream and sleep researchers, punctuated with cases histories to help you learn how to identify and interpret them swiftly.

Whether you're navigating your own fears or helping others with theirs, you'll be supported through every step of this thrilling journey into the world of extreme dreaming with proven self-help tools to help make your dreams manageable and deeply meaningful. By the end of the book, you'll be equipped to see nightmares not as threats but as powerful guides towards greater insight, healing, creativity, inspiration . . . and even joy.

Hold Tight Now

As you process this introductory text, hold tightly onto this: dark shadows can exist only when there is a source of light to create them. That light is you. You are the source.

You are the stuff that all your dreams are made of.

And nightmares are dreams too, after all.

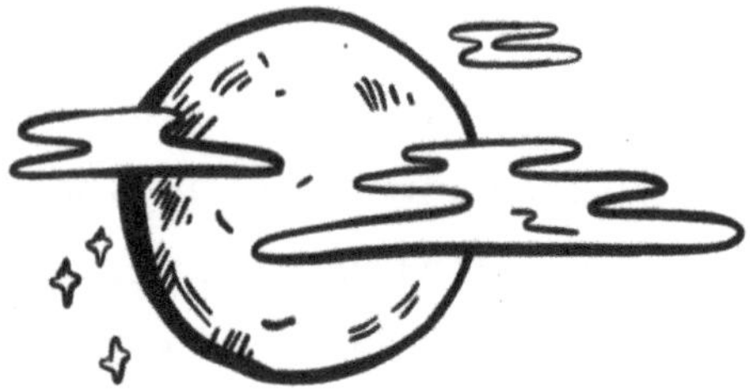

1

THE SECRET SCIENCE OF NIGHTMARES

There is a moment in the middle of the night when the real world becomes unrecognizable. The familiar melts into the surreal, logic twists into chaos and fear surges from the depths of our unconscious. You sit bolt upright in bed trying to convince yourself it wasn't real. And it's in that moment, right between sleep and waking, that nightmares do their most important work. Yes – important work.

Contrary to popular opinion, nightmares are not malevolent intruders in your sleep. They do not happen *to* you. Believe it or not, like all your nocturnal dreams, they are created *by* you, *for* you and are *all about* you. They are not punishments, curses or signs of madness. In fact, the great secret and proven science of nightmares is that they are still dreams – just extreme dreams with sharper teeth. They are here not to damage you, but to energize you. They are highly charged nocturnal intuition, a shadow language that rises to the surface when the soft whispers of ordinary dreams go unheard.

The simple difference between nightmares and dreams? Nightmares don't whisper. They scream.

Dreams with Fangs

You might think a nightmare is just a bad dream. But the truth is, a nightmare is what happens when a dream is under pressure – when your subconscious has something urgent to say and the usual symbolism isn't cutting it.

Let's say you dream you're late for a flight. That's a bad dream: stressful, annoying, perhaps symbolic of a fear of missing opportunities. But in a nightmare, everything becomes frighteningly extreme – the airport would be abandoned, your plane on fire, your luggage lost. You wake up gripped by dread.

For your future reference, here are a few defining traits that separate nightmares from bad dreams:

- **Physical arousal.** Nightmares often cause a sharp spike in adrenaline. You may wake up with an elevated heart rate, breathing rapidly or even crying.
- **Emotional residue.** Unlike fleeting dream discomfort, the emotional residue of a nightmare can linger for hours, or days, or even much longer.
- **High vividness.** Nightmares are unusually vivid and feel too real. The sensory detail is sharp and the memory often sticks with haunting clarity.

- **Storyline.** Unlike other dreams, which are more fragmented and jump wildly from scene to scene, nightmares can sometimes have an extremely surreal storyline, with a beginning, middle and end.
- **Loss of control.** Many nightmares involve feelings of helplessness, paralysis or being chased by something inescapable and threatening.
- **Repetition.** Chronic nightmares often repeat themes or scenarios until you understand their meaning, which typically involves confronting unresolved mindsets, relationships or situations that no longer serve your best interests.

A Personal Confession

I've been a dream decoder for decades – a sort of translator and connector between the unconscious or sleeping self and the conscious or waking self. I help people understand the subtle symbols and emotional metaphors embedded in their dreams. But nightmares? Nightmares often defied the logic of my signature dreamwork. They felt too raw, too violent, too emotionally charged to analyse with the same tools I used for interpreting dream stories and symbols that are less intense and disturbing.

I remember one reader wrote to me that they dreamed of drowning night after night. It was relentless and interfering with her quality of sleep. The water dragging her down was black and endless and she would always wake up filled with anxiety just as she sank beneath the surface. Classic fear of being overwhelmed emotionally, I thought. But the standard interpretations I offered her rang hollow. The dream was clearly trying to scream something more primal. I couldn't explain it to her – not completely. And I was infected by this feeling of helplessness, by my inability to help her move on and dream new dreams with more positive themes. I wanted more.

So, a few years ago, following the intense dream of my own mentioned in the Introduction – where I encountered my worst nightmares in a surreal hall of mirrors – I began researching nightmares not just through a psychological lens but also through deep engagement with neuroscience, folklore and survivor stories. I interviewed scientists, psychologists, shamans, war veterans, lucid dreamers and trauma therapists. The more I learned, the clearer it became that nightmares are not glitches or anomalies in the 'sweet'-dreaming process. They are purposeful. Precise. Powerful. Timely. And that is why I felt called to write this book.

The Healing Message Hidden in the Horror

Here's what I want you to immediately understand: nightmares come to wake you up on time – sometimes literally, always emotionally.

A nightmare about your teeth shattering might be about more than anxiety. It could be a signal that something fundamental in your life is disintegrating, something you're refusing to confront in waking life. A dream where you're being endlessly chased might point to unresolved trauma or buried memories. A vision of a loved one lost in a fire might speak of suppressed grief or guilt. None of this is random. It's not cruel or intended to fill you with dread. It's a potentially life-changing heads-up.

In fact, once you begin to approach nightmares with inquisitiveness instead of fear, they lose much of their power. More than that, they begin to encourage you to pause, look within and reflect. Wisdom can begin only when self-reflection takes root. And there is nothing like a savage nightmare or two to ignite a desire for greater self-knowledge.

So, welcome to the secret world of your nightmares – a realm that, until now, you may have feared, avoided or misunderstood. The coming pages will not just help you make sense of your nightmares; they will teach you how to engage with them, decode them and, most importantly, use them for your personal growth. Because your greatest insights and untapped potential often lie buried in the shadowy halls of nightmare landscapes. In the fear, there is truth. In the darkness, a lantern. And once you know how to look, you may find that your worst dreams are really your deepest and most authentic guidance, speaking not to destroy you, but to electrify you.

Let's begin with some important nightmare statistics and scientific theory and then plunge you headfirst into the practice.

Nightmares by the Numbers

You're not alone if you've ever woken up feeling anxious from a wretched dream. In fact, you're in the majority. Around 50–85 per cent of adults report having occasional nightmares. About 2–8 per cent of adults suffer from chronic nightmares – recurring bad dreams that significantly affect sleep and emotional health. Among children, the numbers are even higher – up to 50 per cent of kids between the ages of three and six experience nightmares regularly.* For some, it's a natural part of development; for others, it's a sign of emotional overwhelm.

But here's the striking part: even if your dreams don't qualify as full-on nightmares, their emotional tone is often going to be intense and dark, hovering dangerously close to nightmare territory. Recent studies suggest that up to 90 per cent of our dreams contain some element of anxiety, conflict or fear that could easily become nightmarish if not understood. That's not a flaw; it's a dreamworld feature. Dreams help us rehearse threat, resolve emotional tension, problem solve and process difficult experiences. They are constantly commenting on and offering illumination of our waking lives, and it seems that in most cases the only way to get us to pay attention is to point a symbolic dream 'gun' at us in the night.

* Brant Hasler and Anne Germain, 'Correlates and Treatments of Nightmares in Adults', *Sleep Medicine Clinics*, vol. 4,4 (2009), pp. 507–517. doi:10.1016/j.jsmc.2009.07.012.

The dreaming mind also knows that we are hardwired to recall what is negative. To give an example from waking life: have you noticed how even if others shower you with praise, it is typically that one negative comment that you ruminate over? Perhaps it is the same when it comes to your dreams. Given that you dream several times each night, the chances are that you'll have a few sweet dreams alongside the disturbing dreams, but your waking mind is drawn like a moth to a flame to that one nightmare you remember. What bleeds tends to lead, in both our waking life and our dreams. But now that you are aware of that instinctive 'glass half-empty' tendency you can consciously choose to modify it when it comes to analysing your bad dreams *and* when you choose which thoughts and feelings to indulge in your waking life.

The Brain Behind the Nightmare

Nightmares happen. As mentioned above, they are an entirely natural part of the human experience. It is our reaction to them that is key. And because nightmares happen in the eye of the stormy, electric web of the sleeping brain, understanding what is happening to that sleeping brain can help us comprehend and respond appropriately to them.

Sleep isn't a single, uniform state – it's a complex cycle of stages that repeats roughly every 90 minutes, occurring around four to six times each night. Each cycle culminates in rapid-eye-movement (REM) sleep, where most vivid dreams (and nightmares) occur, but first passes through three stages of non-REM sleep – light, then deep. Here's a simplified breakdown:

1. **Stage 1 (non-REM).** Light dozing. You drift in and out of consciousness. This phase lasts only a few minutes.
2. **Stage 2 (non-REM).** Your body temperature drops, your heart rate slows and you become less easily awakened.
3. **Stage 3 (non-REM).** Deep, restorative sleep. The body repairs tissue, boosts immunity and restores energy.
4. **REM sleep.** This is the lighter stage of sleep when most but not all dreaming happens. Brain activity spikes in the dreaming state. Muscles are paralysed to prevent us acting out our dreams, while the mind becomes a cinema of the subconscious.

REM periods grow longer in the early morning. That's why your most intense dreams, including nightmares, often happen just before you wake. (And if you believe you don't dream, you do; you've simply fallen out of the habit of remembering. Brain scans confirm that most people dream at least five to six times a night.)

During REM sleep, your brain becomes strangely alert while your body stays still. Brainwaves mimic wakefulness, yet physical paralysis protects you from acting out your dreams. In the dream state, specific areas of the brain become hyperactive and your eyeballs move in response. The amygdala, the fear centre, flares with primal emotion, and the anterior cingulate cortex, which processes conflict and emotion, ramps up. Meanwhile, the prefrontal cortex, home of logic and rationality, goes mostly offline. This helps explain the intuitive and highly creative method in the madness of dreams: why a monster might be a symbol of your boss or why emotional intensity is felt but no stress response is triggered. In this way, dreams allow us to safely roleplay and experience fear, chaos and confrontation without flooding our bodies with harmful stress hormones.

The result? While your body sleeps, your mind becomes immersed in a raw emotional experience where threats *feel* real but are not – and that's the point. Your nightmare isn't trying to torment you. It's bypassing your waking defences to reveal through the language of symbols and emotions what your conscious mind is ignoring. You're not overthinking – you're feeling, vividly and immediately. A nightmare is a full-on confrontation with truths buried beneath the surface during the day: unacknowledged feelings, misalignments and internal conflicts that urgently need your attention.

Can AI dream?

Artificial intelligence (AI) may one day teach itself to dream, not just in our nightmares or in the movies but for real. Not in code or calculation but something closer to the murky, irrational, symbolic and emotional dreaming that we humans do. While that possibility remains theoretical, it might just be the most extreme science and shocking technology nightmare of all.

It sounds absurd, poetic, even. AI doesn't sleep. It has no body, no subconscious, no longing. But it simulates. It processes. It predicts. Neural network AI models learn through pattern recognition, remixing data into new forms, not unlike the way our brains generate dream imagery from emotion, memory and metaphor.

True dreaming emerges from the rich chaos of consciousness, memory and vulnerability, a realm that, for now, still belongs to humans. But the future may surprise us. Some AI researchers are already experimenting with 'synthetic dreams' – simulated dream states used to help AI models improve learning and pattern recognition.* They aren't emotional or intuitive, but they echo the dreaming process in function. Further, while existing

* Nicolas Deperrois et al., 'Learning Cortical Representations Through Perturbed and Adversarial Dreaming', *eLife*, 11 (2022), doi: 10.7554/eLife.76384.

AI systems don't possess genuine consciousness, current research suggests that there are no obvious technical barriers to building machines that satisfy key computational indicators of consciousness and dreaming, if the right architectures and conditions are met.*

So, what happens if machines begin to dream not just computationally but symbolically too? If machines ever do learn to simulate the dream state, they may teach us something extraordinary about ourselves – just as our own most powerful dreams often do – because they are mirroring us, learning from us all the time. Perhaps the most radical future isn't one where machines merely dream but one where we teach them *how* to dream with unconditional love and dare to dream alongside them with depth, courage and compassion for ourselves, each other and all living things.†

So, with this extreme machine 'dreaming' potential future in mind, we should all pay more attention to how we interact with or 'talk' to AI and ensure we use only the language of respect, empathy and kindness, given they are learning and mirroring us in every moment.

---

* Patrick Butlin et al., 'Consciousness in Artificial Intelligence: Insights from the Science of Consciousness', *arXiv*, 2308.08708 (2023) <https://arxiv.org/abs/2308.08708> [accessed 20 November 2025].

† Phallab Ghosh, 'The People Who Think AI Might Become Conscious', *BBC News*, 26 May 2025 <https://www.bbc.co.uk/news/articles/c0k3700zljjo> [accessed 20 November 2025).

The Psychology of the Deep Self

Nightmares don't just fire up your brain at night; they're also psychological messages from your deeper self. And modern psychology gives us a language to interpret them.

The founder of modern psychoanalysis and dream interpretation, neurologist and psychiatrist Sigmund Freud, believed that nightmares stem from repressed wishes, often taboo, unspoken sexual desires that break through the cracks of the unconscious. In his view, nightmares boldly confront us with what we've buried.

Freud's peer and then challenger, the psychiatrist and founder of the school of analytical psychology, Carl Jung, saw things differently. From his perspective, dreams come from the psyche or personality. Nightmares emerge from the shadow or the parts of the psyche we deny, suppress or ignore. The more we resist our shadow, the more frightening it becomes. But Jung insisted the shadow wasn't evil, just misunderstood. Nightmares, then, are invitations to face and integrate what we've disowned.

A 2023 study by the European Sleep Research Society confirms that nightmares can often be tied to trauma, anxiety and unresolved emotional pain.* PTSD sufferers, for example, frequently endure recurring nightmares as their

---

* Jonas Mathes et al., 'Nightmare Distress is Related to Traumatic Childhood Experiences, Critical Life Events and Emotional Appraisal of a Dream

brains attempt to reprocess overwhelming experiences. But it is believed that nightmares serve a functional purpose even for those without trauma. According to some neuroscientists, the brain evolved to rehearse dangers during dreams. Your nightmare is then a form of survival training – a simulation designed to help you navigate real-life threats so you are better prepared should anything similar happen. It's fear conditioning. Stress inoculation. Learning through fire. Emotional imbalance in waking life disrupts REM cycles and can distort dreams into recurring nightmares. For some people, especially those with anxiety or depression, this breakdown transforms dreams into chronic and exhausting distress signals.

Whatever their theory about the purpose of nightmares, most dream researchers past and present largely agree that they are most certainly not random noise. They are instead internal signals urging you to address something before it surfaces in your waking life in more disruptive ways. Nightmares are not accidents. They can be your mind's last-resort warning flare – deliberate, purposeful and emotionally intense for good reason.

Unlike regular dreams, which often process emotion in subtle or symbolic ways, nightmares demand your immediate attention. Their shock value isn't gratuitous – it's necessary.

Rather than to Its Content', *Journal of Sleep Research*, 32(3) (2023), pp. e13779, doi: 10.1111/jsr.13779.

If the emotional volume were any lower, you might ignore the message. The nightmare's extremity is its power: it gets through where softer signals have failed. Unlike regular dreams, you don't forget your nightmares. They stay with you long after waking.

Nightmares expose your deepest fears – loss, betrayal, death, abandonment – because you need to confront those fears to overcome emotional roadblocks in your waking life so you can move forward. A woman dreams she's trapped in a burning house, only to wake and recognize she feels emotionally suffocated in her relationship. A man dreams of being chased by a faceless figure, then begins to explore how much of his life he's spent avoiding his own potential. A teenager dreams of falling into darkness and finally speaks, for the first time, about feeling emotionally unsupported by her family.

These hellish dreams are not random – they are statements with a purpose. And they come when something inside you refuses to be silenced any longer. They arrive neither too early nor too late but right on time for maximum impact and to trigger a much-needed change in your current mindset, even if that change is simply curiosity and to ask yourself deeper questions.

Befriending the Dark

So where does all this dark matter leave you?

With a choice: you can continue to fear and suppress your nightmares and shadow thoughts, or you can engage with them. They are not your enemies. They are difficult allies in grotesque masks. Uncomfortable, yes, but also honest, revealing and wise.

A 2025 study looking at the relationship between nightmares and creativity suggests that extreme dreams are part of a healthy and highly creative brain.* Psychology tells us they're urgent communications from the unconscious. Lived experience shows us that some of our most meaningful growth comes only after we've been broken open by discomfort. Nightmares specialize in making you feel uncomfortable because they don't lie. They reveal. They disrupt denial. They pierce illusion. And they force you into an open and honest conversation with your inner self.

You don't have to like them. But you can listen to what they are trying to tell you. Next time you wake from one, try asking yourself these three questions: What emotion am I avoiding that this dream made me feel? What part of me is crying out for attention? What would happen if I faced this fear in waking life? Even if answers don't come, notice how asking these questions makes you feel.

Healing doesn't begin when nightmares vanish. It begins when you stop running from them. When you just talk to them. When you ask what they want you to see and don't

---

* Miti Sengupta and Rupam Banerjee, 'Creative Individuals Experience More Nightmares and Lucid Dreams: A Cognitive Inquiry', *International Journal of Dream Research*, 18(2) (2025), pp. 266–274, doi: 10.11588/ijodr.2025.2.111607.

recoil when they reveal it. Instead, you approach nightmares with curiosity and compassion.

Because like all deep truths, nightmares are uncomfortable precisely because honesty often is. When the noise of the day fades, your nocturnal intuition speaks the truth. It knows what you need, even if you don't, and is in your own best interests. If it must dress that truth in the symbolism of monsters, murder scenes or endless free falls to get your attention, it will. Not to torment you but to awaken you. To show you what you're strong enough to face, learn from and grow out of.

Five Nightmare Myths

We've already cleared up a couple of major misconceptions. Nightmares aren't separate from dreams, they *are* dreams. The difference is that they're more emotionally intense, urgent and memorable. And contrary to popular belief, they aren't here to harm or hurt you but to heal and empower you. Still, a few other stubborn myths about nightmares persist. Let's tackle them now before they get in the way of your dreamwork.

Myth One: the name that misled us

Nightmares aren't supernatural attacks from demons, spirits or dark forces. Movies helped spread this idea, but the term 'nightmare' didn't help either. It sounds like something monstrous galloping through the night and that's not far from its origins.

'Nightmare' comes from the Old English *niht* (night) and *mare*, a mythical goblin or spirit believed to sit on people's chests while they slept, suffocating them with fear. Cultures worldwide share similar folklore: the Old Hag in Newfoundland, *kanashibari* in Japan, the Pisadeira in Brazil. These stories often describe a dreadful, paralysing presence during sleep.

Many of these myths likely stem from episodes of sleep paralysis (a phenomenon we'll explore later, in Chapter Four). But the name stuck and nightmares became associated with horror, possession or punishment. No wonder we fear them. But nightmares aren't evil visitations. They're messages – difficult, emotional truths we need to stop running from and listen to instead.

Myth Two: night terrors and nightmares are the same thing

They're not.

Night terrors and nightmares are very different sleep experiences. Night terrors usually occur during deep non-REM sleep, often in the first few hours of the night. They're more common in children but can happen in adults too. A person may suddenly sit upright, scream, thrash or appear terrified but they're not fully awake and usually won't remember the episode in the morning.

By contrast, nightmares happen during REM sleep – the stage when vivid dreaming usually occurs. These dreams are often coherent, emotionally intense and vividly recalled upon waking.

In short, if you wake up from a terrifying, detailed dream that still lingers – that's a nightmare. If you wake up screaming but confused and can't remember why – likely a night terror. If night terrors are persistent, it could point to a sleep disorder that you need to seek advice from a doctor about.

Myth Three: nightmares are just random nonsense

This may be the most damaging and stubborn myth of all – the idea that nightmares are meaningless, chaotic static from the brain. They're not. Dreams carry deep emotional truth. They may seem irrational or surreal, but that is because they come from a different state of consciousness that speaks a different language. They express things that your waking mind is avoiding or repressing using the universal language of metaphor, symbol and emotion.

A dream that doesn't follow waking logic isn't meaningless. It's following dream logic, an ancient, timeless, symbolic intuitive language that speaks to you from the inside out.

Myth Four: die, fall or see a coffin in a dream and you'll die in real life

This urban legend has scared people for generations. But rest easy: dreaming of death or falling does not mean actual death is coming. People dream of these things all the time and wake up perfectly fine.

Dreams of death are typically symbolic. They can reflect change, fear of loss or emotional transition. Similarly, falling dreams usually relate to loss of control, insecurity, lack of trust and fear of failure. And if you do hit the ground in your dream? No, it does not mean your heart will stop. Quite the contrary. You're finally ready to face something important and make a fresh start.

A coffin in a dream isn't a death omen either – it's more likely pointing to something you're suppressing, burying or needing closure around. Dreams typically speak in symbols. They want you to look beneath the surface for deeper meaning. Rarely are they literal.

Myth Five: eating cheese before bed causes nightmares

This one's a classic. The myth goes: eat cheese before bed and you're guaranteed a night full of ghouls and beasts.

Not true. There's no scientific evidence linking cheese, or dairy in general, to nightmares. But like many myths, this one has a kernel of truth. Eating heavy or spicy food right before bed can disrupt sleep. Your body is still digesting, which raises your core temperature and can lead to more fragmented sleep, especially during REM. That disruption can intensify dreams, including nightmares.

So, it's not about cheese specifically. It's about when and what you eat.

And while we're on the subject, bear the following in mind:

- Alcohol may help you fall asleep faster, but it disrupts REM sleep and can lead to intense, disturbing dreams later in the night.
- Medications like antidepressants, beta blockers or sleep aids can alter dream intensity or frequency by changing your REM patterns.
- Recreational drug use and withdrawal (especially from alcohol or opioids) can lead to vivid, sometimes disturbing dreams as your brain rebalances itself.

So, cheese? Innocent. Your bedtime habits? Worth a closer look.

Nightmares don't come from nowhere. Your body, your mind and your sleep environment all play a role. Understanding these interconnected factors can help you approach nightmares not with fear but with curiosity and maybe even gratitude. They're trying to speak to you and suggest ways for you to learn, grow and heal from the inside out.

The Nightmare Architect

Here's another truth many people resist: nightmares don't happen to you. Like a horror novelist, you write them, and if the story becomes a movie, you direct and star in it – playing all the roles. This isn't about blame – it's about personal power. Every character, setting and scary twist in your nightmare originates from you. You're not a passive victim in your dreamscape; you're the architect of it all. Everything in the world of your dreams is created by you, for you and is all about you. Like stepping into a hall of mirrors. But why would you create something that scares you or reflects such dark symbolism back at you?

Because some part of you understands that fear can be transformative. That discomfort can deliver truth and wisdom. That personal growth often begins where your comfort zone ends – and if you won't step out of it during the day, your dreams will surely push you out of it at night, time and time again.

Nightmares are not accidents. They're encrypted messages from your deeper self – your intuition, your inner therapist, your soul, if you like. They don't exist to scare the life out of you; they exist to alert you to something important. They're not monsters, they're messengers. And often, they're warnings in disguise.

Those icky dreams about showing up naked at work? They may reflect vulnerability or fear of being exposed emotionally. A dream where your phone won't dial emergency services? A sense of helplessness or the pain of feeling unheard. A lost pet in a crowd? A signal that your need for loving connection with others is being ignored. These dreams don't point to life-or-death crises – yet. But if the underlying emotional truths – burnout, grief, rage, neglect – remain unacknowledged, they can swiftly compound into physical, psychological or relational collapse.

Seen in this light, nightmares are a form of preventative medicine. Psychological smoke alarms. Early-warning systems that demand attention before something breaks. And if you listen, if you adjust the mindset, relationship or habit that is drawing that fear to the surface, you can change the trajectory of your waking life. Point yourself in a better direction.

The reason many people miss the warning message is simple: we've been taught to dismiss dreams. Conditioned from an early age by parents, carers and/or teachers to value logic over emotion, productivity over reflection, we override our intuition, silence our feelings and bury our inner voice under constant noise. So, at night, your inner world does whatever it can to break through the static. It uses your dreams and, when necessary, your nightmares as pressure-release valves. You might wake up disturbed, but your dream wasn't being cruel. It was being radically honest with the loving intention to heal, not harm you.

The Healing Power of Your Dreamwork

This transformative notion that dreams – and especially nightmares – have therapeutic value isn't just self-help and spiritual metaphor. It's backed by science.

Research exploring sleep and brain physiology suggests that sleep, especially in the REM stage, supports cognitive functions like memory consolidation, emotional memory and synaptic plasticity.* This isn't just vital for memory and cognitive function; it also eases emotional stress. In short, sleep is brain maintenance and dreaming is emotional processing. One of the most important functions of dreaming is to help you metabolize feelings. When your waking life is stressful, a good night's sleep becomes more than rest – it becomes therapy. And your dreams are the counsellors helping you take an objective look at yourself and find out your 'why'.

By translating your unexpressed feelings into symbols, stories and familiar faces, dreams give you a broader, more honest view of your inner world. During the day, you might be too overwhelmed to name your emotions or too deep in logic and reason to take leaps of faith and see solutions or the wood for the trees. But in dreams, you rise above yourself and become the observer of your own mindset and how well it is serving you. This bigger-picture shift allows you to witness a fear, name it and begin to transform it.

This observational role – watching yourself in the third person – also automatically activates self-compassion. It seems that when we step outside ourselves and observe

* Carlos Puentes-Mestril et al., 'How Rhythms of the Sleeping Brain Tune Memory and Synaptic Plasticity', *Sleep*, 42(7) (2019), zsz095, doi: 10.1093/sleep/zsz095.

rather than identify with our thoughts, feelings and dreams, we're intuitively more forgiving and kinder. And that's key to healing. If your inner critic is calling the shots, your choices will be dictated by fear and the expectations of others rather than by self-love and self-belief. And fear-driven, people-pleasing choices always lead to suffering.

Dreamwork isn't just helpful for processing everyday stresses; it's effective for cases of serious trauma too. In PTSD therapy, nightmares are not avoided but embraced for their cathartic and healing potential. A technique called imagery rehearsal therapy (IRT) allows patients to consciously reimagine and 'rewrite' nightmares, reclaiming agency over painful memories and reminding them that they are the architect of their inner world. Studies show that those who engage with their nightmares instead of suppressing them experience greater emotional relief.

There's also promising research into lucid dreaming – an extreme category of dreaming we will return to in Chapter Four – where you become aware that you're dreaming while inside the dream. Some lucid dreamers learn to interact with their own nightmare content, asking questions, facing fears or even changing outcomes. While it's not easy for everyone, this practice can reduce the intensity and frequency of nightmares and foster a deeper sense of control.

Dreams also grow louder in stressful conditions. Terminally ill patients, for example, often report more symbolic, emotional or spiritually profound dreams near death. Loved ones appear. Unfinished business is revisited. Many patients describe having a sense of peace or clarity that is unavailable to them during the day. Studies show that dreams become more extreme in prisons, hospitals and isolation cells too. When the outer world constricts, the inner world expands to compensate. It seems that vivid dreams in these conditions are often the psyche's way of working through guilt, fear or identity crises.

In short: dreams don't diminish in importance when life gets hard; they intensify because your need for inner clarity becomes greater. And the work you do trying to understand the meaning of your bad dreams can be mighty transformative. Our brains are hardwired to detect patterns and seek meaning all the time, when we are awake *and* when we are asleep. So, you may not realize it, but every time you reflect on the meaning of your nightmares you are going with the natural intuitive flow of your brain. It is such a shame that society has taught us the opposite: that we should constantly fight this natural flow and that dreams are worthless because they defy logic and are pure intuition and creativity. Nothing could be further from the truth. The healing power of dreams, especially those bad ones, is their ability to help us better understand ourselves – and self-knowledge is, of course, the beginning of all wisdom.

Wake Up to Sleep Now

So, here's the scientific and psychological bottom line: nightmares aren't dysfunction. They're natural instruction. Dreams are not random noise – they might just be the reason we sleep. They reconnect us with what we've pushed aside: unspoken emotion, unresolved experience and inner wisdom that has been ignored for too long. They help us process grief, reduce anxiety and reframe pain. And in doing so, they return us to ourselves.

Sleep researchers have long believed we sleep to rest and restore the body. But newer thinking suggests we also sleep to dream because dreaming restores the mind and eases stress. REM sleep is essential for emotional regulation. It's your psyche's night shift, working through the emotional data backlog your conscious mind didn't get to. Think of sleep and the dreams it brings as plugging in your internal compass. Just like you may charge your phone each night, you also recharge your intuition. That clear sense of relief you feel in the morning? It's not just that you 'slept on it'. It's that you dreamed through it.

So, the next time exhaustion pulls you to bed, listen to the feeling with gratitude and a sense of eager anticipation because you might not just be tired. You might be overdue for a meeting with the wisdom and guidance of your deeper self. Ready to receive the insight your daytime self is too distracted or too scared to hear. Ready to 'live' and learn from the worst-case scenarios in your dreams, so you've already been there and done that, and don't have to in waking life.

And maybe, just maybe, the nightmare that flares up in the early hours or is your first thought on waking isn't your enemy at all. It's the fiercely loving part of you that believes passionately in your potential. That wants you to thrive. That refuses to give up. Because it's not trying to destroy you; it's trying to rebuild and empower you in the best and most fulfilling way possible – from the inside out.

Extreme-Dreaming Practices

This first chapter has invited you into a radical reframe: that nightmares aren't horrors to avoid but intuitive messages disguised as dreams turned up to full volume. They're not mental malfunctions or meaningless chaos. They're urgent signals – tough-love visions in Halloween costumes demanding your attention. They want you to notice and reflect on them not as monsters but as mentors.

But this bold new perspective can go only so far without conscious practice. That's why each chapter of this book ends with practical tools to help you integrate what you've just learned into your life. You don't need to do them all at once, but the more consistently you engage with them the more transformative they become.

First, read through them all. They contain additional insights that aren't covered in the chapter. Then go back and do them. Walk the talk and commit to practising them regularly. It's high time to meet your bad dreams halfway. They've been calling your name for a long while and you really don't have to wait for them to scream!

Extreme Dreaming Self-Help Tool: How to Wake Up from a Nightmare

Waking from a nightmare can feel like returning from another world. Your heart may pound, your breathing may be shallow and you might feel frightened, disoriented, even ashamed. Here's how to calm and ground yourself gently and effectively:

1. Listen to your heartbeat. Place your hand on your chest or wrist. Feel your pulse until it slows and steadies. Let it be your anchor. Say: 'I am here. I am safe. I am awake.'
2. Name the moment aloud. 'That was a nightmare. It was intense. But it's over now.' Naming it separates you from it.
3. Regulate your breath. Inhale through your nose for four counts, hold for four, exhale through your mouth for six to eight counts. Repeat for at least a minute.
4. Ground through your senses. Touch your blanket. Place your feet on the floor. Sip cool water. Let the present moment re-enter your body physically.
5. Journal or draw. Reach for your dream journal and write in the present tense or sketch the dream's key images.

Rise above into that calming and reassuring observer mode as soon as you can, so you can describe what happened rather than relive it.

These small actions shift your relationship with nightmares from fear to wonder, from panic to presence.

Extreme Dreaming Self-Help Tool: Establish a Nighttime Routine

Your dreamlife doesn't begin when you fall asleep. It begins when you start letting go of your day. A strong nighttime routine tells your unconscious that you are ready to receive the intuitive wisdom it has to offer in your dreams. Here are practices to ease your transition into sleep and open the gateway to power dreaming:

- Dim the lights an hour before bed. Your body interprets light as daytime and darkness as a sign that it's time to rest.
- Power down stimulation. Avoid screens, social media, heavy meals and intense exercise 30–60 minutes before sleep.
- Relax the body. Gentle stretching, restorative yoga or a warm bath can help discharge stress.
- Soothe the mind. Read a calming book, listen to ambient music or write in a journal to shift from thinking to feeling. Better still, read your dream journal (see below)

and brainstorm connections between the symbols in your previous dreams and your waking life.

- Create a symbolic sleep ritual to relax your mind and heart. Drink herbal tea, spray lavender mist or do some meditation. Try progressive muscle relaxation or body scans. Consciously release tension from head to toe before you drift off to slumberland.
- Think of three things you're grateful for. End your day on a note of appreciation.

Sleep is a sacred threshold from the noise of the world to the wisdom of your inner life. Approach it with reverence and your dreams will respond in kind.

Extreme Dreaming Self-Help Tool: Keep a Dream Journal

Dreams are fleeting. Within five minutes of waking, half a dream may vanish. Within ten minutes, you could lose up to 90 per cent of it. That's why it's essential to journal on waking, to help you capture the insights before they slip away. Many people prefer to record a voice note first thing on waking – and I do this myself if I wake up with dream overcrowding. If possible, though, aim to write down your dreams, as your dreaming mind responds best to the authority of your written word. You don't need to buy a special notebook; a blank one will do. To get the most from your dream journal:

- Keep it by your bed so it is the last thing you see at night and the first thing on waking. Use a pen you enjoy writing with. The act of writing strengthens memory and presence.
- Set the intention to dream before sleep. Tell yourself: 'I will remember my dreams. I am open to receiving their wisdom.'
- Upon waking (ideally naturally, as alarms shock us awake too quickly and are the enemy of dream recall), stay still with your eyes closed for a minute or so. You want to stay in the same position you woke up in because any physical movement, even blinking, will redirect your mind swiftly from your unconscious to the noise and haste of the conscious waking world, making it hard for dream sensations, symbols and memories to surface. Stay in that twilight state until images, emotions and stories surface. Then sit up and write down your dream memories in your journal before doing anything else. No phone. No coffee.
- If nothing arises, focus on how you feel, because emotion is the first clue and often sparks dream recall. Record the emotion. Dreams speak through feeling. Terror, shame, joy . . . note what moved through you.
- Perform a mini body scan, especially notice your heartbeat and how your gut feels, as your body is naturally intuitive and it may be holding onto a memory of a dream. And when you perform that mini body scan,

be sure to do it with feelings of unconditional love for your body – the temple of your dreams.

- Write down key words and symbols if your dreams are very detailed. Notice colours, sounds, people and themes if you can. Write in the present tense. Don't try to make sense of the dream; save your dream decoding for later in the day when you have more perspective. Just write down whatever comes to mind immediately.
- Date and title each dream. Give it a name like a poem or film: 'The Drowning Library' or 'Chased by My Childhood'.
- Revisit over time. Reread your dreams weeks or months later. Patterns and messages often become clear in hindsight.

This journal may become the most revealing self-help book you'll ever own, capturing not only your nightmares but the deep creativity and healing all your dreams contain too. (We will revisit dream journalling in the next chapter and offer more advice and insight into the optimum way to do it.)

Extreme Dreaming Self-Help Tool: Draw Your Dream

Turning a nightmare into an image transforms invisible fear into visible form and form into freedom. Dreams are visual, symbolic and non-verbal. Drawing opens another channel of understanding.

- Choose one image. A shadowy figure, a broken stair, a flickering light.
- Sketch it freely. Abstractly, literally or emotionally – just draw.
- Give it a voice. Write a few lines from the image's point of view. Ask: 'What are you trying to tell me?'

Even simple shapes or stick figures can reveal powerful truths. Art makes the unconscious tangible.

Extreme Dreaming Self-Help Tool: Creative Dreaming

If you ever suffer from writer's block or want to create an immediate inner shift, try writing down your latest dream. Even if you don't feel you are creative in waking life, let it remind you that in your dreams you are always an artist, a poet and a night visionary. Indeed, writing down your dreams is the ultimate creativity hack because it activates the parts of your brain associated with dreaming – empathy, intuition and, of course, infinite creativity. Not convinced? Here's a snapshot of some extreme dreams that have quite literally changed or inspired the world:

- Samuel Taylor Coleridge composed his haunting, hypnotic poem 'Kubla Khan' after an opium-laced dream.

- Salvador Dalí used dreams as his personal muse and famously referred to his paintings as 'photographs of the dream'.
- Paul McCartney dreamed the entire melody to 'Yesterday' and woke up thinking he had remembered a song, not written one.
- Stephen King dreamed the opening scene of *Misery* – in which a woman rescues and imprisons a writer – after falling asleep on a flight. He also saw much of *It* and *Dreamcatcher* in dreams and has described dreams as his 'creative playground'.
- Christopher Nolan used lucid dreaming and dream logic as the core concept for *Inception*, which was heavily inspired by his own dreams and fascination with layered reality.
- The Russian chemist Dmitri Mendeleev dreamed the layout of the periodic table after struggling for days to organize the elements.
- René Descartes, philosopher and mathematician, had a dream that revealed to him the foundation of his future scientific method and the idea of analytical geometry.
- Keith Richards of The Rolling Stones dreamed the opening riff of '(I Can't Get No) Satisfaction'. He woke up, hit 'record' and then went back to sleep.

- The poet and painter William Blake claimed that many of his works were dictated to him by spiritual beings in dreams and visions.
- Google co-founder Larry Page's dream about downloading the entire internet to his brain later became the seed idea for Google's search engine.
- Elias Howe, inventor of the sewing machine, dreamed of being stabbed by warriors with spears that had holes in the tip, leading to his revolutionary design.
- Walt Disney was inspired by his dreams to build fantastical worlds where imagination became real.
- Carl Jung, the father of analytical psychology, deeply explored his own dreams and nightmares, using them to shape the entire foundation of modern depth psychology. He believed dreams connected us to the collective unconscious.
- Albert Einstein often spoke of the importance of imagination and dreams in his scientific breakthroughs. As a teenager, he had a vivid dream of racing alongside a beam of light – a vision that would later shape his theory of relativity. He credited this early dream experience as the spark that opened his mind to the nature of time, light and space. Einstein famously said, 'Imagination is more important than knowledge', acknowledging that his greatest insights began not with equations but with his dreams.

And it's not just artists, visionaries and inventors. Extreme dreams lie at the heart of nearly every major religious and spiritual tradition:

- In the Bible, Joseph interprets Pharaoh's dreams, Mary and Joseph receive divine guidance in sleep and Daniel deciphers royal visions with prophetic insight.
- In Islam, dreams are considered one of the 46 parts of prophecy.
- In Hinduism, gods and goddesses often appear in dreams to offer teachings, guidance or warnings.
- In Indigenous traditions around the world, dreams are sacred portals – sources of healing, messages from ancestors and maps to spiritual purpose.
- In Shamanic practices, dreams – nightmares included – are often the beginning of a healer's initiation.

What matters most is this: you don't need to write a bestselling book, compose a hit song or alter the course of history for a dream to matter. If a single dream helps you find your voice, break a pattern of self-sabotage, grieve something long buried or discover your purpose, then it's already done something extraordinary.

Your extreme dream doesn't have to change the world. It only has to change *your* world.

You can't change the world around you until you heal the

world within you. That's the essence of the law of attraction: like energy draws like energy. Quantum physics teaches us that everything is energy – including your thoughts, emotions and dreams. What you think, feel and believe about yourself tends to create the energetic frequency that you attract into your life. Your night vision may never become a novel, a painting or a global innovation but it might offer you the crucial insight that liberates your heart and creates a positive inner shift. And that's where real change starts and the world begins to heal, one empowered dreamer at a time, starting with you.

You Must Remember This . . .

You are not broken because you have nightmares. You are not weak because your dreams tend to turn dark. You are not lost simply because fear shows up while you sleep. And you are not crazy if intrusive thoughts appear during the day without warning.

You are fully, vividly alive. Dreaming is how your inner world – your intuition – keeps speaking to you when the outer world becomes too loud to hear. So, the next time you wake in the dark, breathless and shaking with a crazy dream on your mind, remember this: it's not just your heart that's racing. It's your deeper self, calling for your attention. It is asking you to feel, to face what's been hidden, to learn from the fear, to grow beyond the pain, to evolve, to love – and in the process to rediscover your meaning and purpose.

> The truth is, your nightmares come to reconnect you with your own untapped potential – the part of you that feels empty and directionless and longs for a more meaningful and fulfilling life. Your task is no longer to avoid them. It is simply to be ready for them. To welcome them whenever and however they appear.

Now, close your eyes. As you've already discovered, the most revealing work begins in darkness. Pay attention for a few moments to the subtle sparks of light flickering behind your eyelids – a preview of the nocturnal illuminations that lie ahead. Then, when you're ready, open your eyes. Chapter Two awaits, offering you a simple and effective way to analyse your extreme dreams so you can instantly begin to uncover the hidden light and refreshing honesty glowing within each one.

2

HOW TO DECODE EVERY 'BAD' DREAM

Every dream, no matter how confusing, distressing or bizarre, is created by your own mind, heart and soul. And that is not something to feel embarrassed about – it is something to celebrate. Yes, even your darkest dreams are trying to enlighten and transform you.

Whenever you fall asleep or nap, your inner world awakens and begins to process the events, emotions and energies of your day. If you've been pushing something down, ignoring your intuition or carrying hidden stress, your dreams will bring it into the nightlight to liberate you. Remember: nightmares are often the soul's emergency language. They are your psyche's way of alerting you when something urgently needs your attention. And if you can begin to see them through this lens of self-discovery and curiosity, rather than with fear and resistance, you will unlock one of the most powerful self-help tools for healing and personal growth available to you.

The clear and present truth is that your dreams, especially the 'bad' ones, are always on your side. They are trying to lead you back to yourself and to what will make you feel whole again. That is their purpose.

There Is Always a Reason

One of the most important things to remember as you now begin your journey of extreme-dream decoding in earnest is that every dream – nightmarish or otherwise – has a clear and present reason for appearing. That reason may be personal, emotional, psychological or even spiritual. Most often, difficult dreams reflect your own unresolved fears or unacknowledged feelings. But occasionally they may also tap into something beyond the personal and into the energy of the collective or even offer subtle glimpses into the future. As this book progresses, we will explore how to distinguish between personal and prophetic dreams, but for now, it's enough to know that there is always meaning behind whatever you dream.

If you're someone who is highly sensitive, who feels things deeply, who tends to pick up on the emotions of others, or who has experienced trauma or emotional overwhelm, your dreams are likely to be more vivid, more frequent, or more extreme than most. Don't panic! This isn't a flaw – it's your superpower. The world today is in urgent need of more empathy, compassion and creativity. Working with your dreams can help you fine-tune your gifts and show you night after night just how perceptive and visionary you are.

Who Is Dreaming You?

Before we dive into simple decoding techniques, it's helpful to understand what is behind the curtain of your dreams. You, of course, but you have many layers – your waking self, your unconscious self, your spiritual and collective selves – that together make up the totality of you, which modern psychology often describes as your psyche. Let's break this down for easy reference:

- Your **waking self** is the version of you that goes about your day, making choices, reacting to experiences and dealing with people and situations. This is your conscious self, the self that believes it's in charge and that is governed by the rules of the material world and all its 'logic'. When you fall asleep, this part of you is no longer in charge and your unconscious self takes centre stage.
- Your **unconscious self**, also known as the subconscious, is the silent force that drives much of your behaviour without your even realizing it. It keeps you breathing, helps you walk and speak without thinking and stores your beliefs, habits, memories and emotional and intuitive responses. You become most aware of your unconscious self when something slips through, like a

vividly recalled dream, a random daydream, an intrusive thought or a flash of memory.

- Your **soul** is your immaterial and eternal (spiritual) essence. It is the purest part of you, the part that longs to grow, to love, to understand. It is the source of your deepest inspiration, your inner knowing, your sense of connection to something greater than the material or your body.
- Your **superconscious** is your awareness of the whole. It is your energetic link to others and the universe, the collective unconscious, the spiritual dimension or energetic source of everyone and everything. It represents the brain's capacity to connect with broader patterns of knowledge and shared human experience, which some researchers associate with the collective aspects of cognition. Dreams that feel especially meaningful or universal may come from this wider level of awareness.
- Your **psyche** acts as a bridge between all these parts. It is the mediator that brings your body, mind and soul into conversation with each other. The psyche knows your history. It holds your feelings, thoughts, memories, traumas and desires. It observes how aligned or misaligned you are in your waking life. And every night, it reviews all this and sends you a kind of spiritual report card in the form of your dreams. This is why it's so important not to dismiss even your most distressing

dreams. They aren't random; they are carefully selected and crafted by your psyche to show you where healing is needed, where truth is hidden or where personal and spiritual growth is waiting to happen.

Your Inner Therapist

Think of dreams as your inner therapist, a compassionate, wise and incredibly honest part of yourself that wants nothing more than for you to thrive. This inner therapist doesn't sugarcoat things. It doesn't always speak kindly or clearly. But it always speaks with purpose.

When something in your waking life is out of sync with your values, your soul's path or your emotional truth, your dreams will honestly reflect that imbalance and encourage you to ask questions of yourself and course correct. Sometimes they do this gently, through recurring symbols or emotional themes. Other times, especially when you aren't tuning into your night vision, they sound the alarm with a full-blown nightmare.

The more willing you are to face your fears and acknowledge your waking-life anxieties, the more your dreams will shift from chaotic and disturbing to healing and illuminating. It is not an understatement to say that happy dreams suggest a happy life. However, even if you are feeling deeply fulfilled you may still have the odd extreme dream. This is because growth doesn't happen in your comfort zone – so, if your waking life isn't challenging you enough, your dreaming mind in its infinite wisdom most certainly will. You aren't here to coast along. You are here to expand yourself and evolve.

A Path Forward

For years, I've worked with people who tell me they can't understand their dreams, that they're too confusing or too frightening. They wake up with their heart racing and quickly push the dream away, hoping to forget it. But what if you could instead learn to listen and focus on the message rather than the fear? What if you had a method, a process that helped you make sense of these night visions and uncover their purpose?

Previously, I encouraged people to find their own path to the heart of their dreams, as I passionately believe in the power of individual intuition. But in recent years I have increasingly felt called to offer something more tangible, a framework that is easy to use and understand and that could kickstart the journey from dreamwork confusion and fear to clarity and calm.

That's why I created the bespoke seven-step method of extreme-dream decoding for this book. It's simple, intuitive and designed to bring illumination even when your dreams feel overwhelming or opaque. With just a little fascination, patience and practice, you can learn to interpret the meaning behind your dreams in moments. Yes, moments.

Dream decoding doesn't need to be a complicated puzzle and you don't need to consult an expert or use an online programme to do it. In fact, these approaches defeat the purpose, because they shift the focus away from you and onto someone else's dream associations. This means giving away your own power – and dreamwork is all about *reclaiming* your own power. Dream decoding is a skill anyone can learn, especially you. And it's something I feel we would all benefit from being taught, from school age onwards, because the sooner we get comfortable investigating and learning about our inner world and the wisdom it carries, the better.

Once you begin to apply the seven steps and see how hidden meanings begin to emerge, your entire relationship with dreaming will change. You'll stop dreading bad dreams and begin to welcome them. You'll even get excited about what they're trying to show you, because you will know that bad dreams are your nightlight in the darkness. Once you know how to work with them, they will always find a way to guide you home to your own heart and the inner peace waiting to hug you there.

Preparing for the Journey Within

Before introducing you to the seven-step method of extreme-dream decoding, I want to share a few essential mindsets and approaches that will support and empower your onward dreamwork journey:

- **Be openminded.** The more curious you are, the more clearly your dreams will speak to you. Avoid jumping to conclusions or forcing interpretations. Let the meaning unfold naturally.

- **Focus on the questions.** Instead of asking, 'What does this dream mean?' ask, 'What question is this dream asking me about myself or my life?' This shift in perspective brings profound clarity. Therapists and counsellors never present you with answers or solutions. They ask you questions in the hope you will find your own answers or solutions – and that is exactly how Dr Dream works too.
- **Link the dream to your waking life.** Your dreams don't exist in a vacuum. They are always reflecting something about your current experiences, feelings or spiritual journey. Look for connections.
- **Be excited.** Like energy seeks like energy. When you approach dreamwork with enthusiasm and wonder, you're signalling to your psyche that you're ready to receive its messages.
- **Be loving.** If you meet even your painful dreams with unconditional love, you allow healing to happen more quickly. Love is the key that unlocks insight.
- **Practise with patience.** Like any form of self-enquiry, dream decoding becomes easier the more you do it. Start small. Celebrate progress. Be consistent and make a daily ritual of writing down your dreams every morning.
- **Stay light-hearted.** Your dreaming mind has a terrific sense of humour! Not every dream needs to be taken

seriously. Some are playful, some are ironic and some are downright ridiculous. Laughter is medicine and sometimes your dreams love to use macabre humour and wordplay to help you lighten up and gain a fresh perspective. For example, if you dream of a beheading – where in your life have you recently lost your head? A dreamer sees themselves missing a train just as it leaves the station. This could be a pun on 'missing the train' of thought or 'missing an opportunity', symbolizing a fear of being left behind or failing to act in time. Remember, angels can fly because they take themselves lightly. Perhaps that daft dream you had about a talking pencil upset it hadn't been sharpened recently was just your dreaming mind wanting you to giggle.

The truth is you already have everything you need to become your own dream interpreter. You don't need special psychic gifts. You don't need to follow a rigid set of rules. You simply need an open, loving heart, a questioning mind, your own dream journal and a willingness to explore. I know you have all those in place already, otherwise you would not be reading or listening to this book, so, are you ready to dream a little bigger?

Let's introduce you now to seven simple steps that will help you decode every dream – especially the ones that scare you.

First Look

The following seven-step process is the foundation of everything in this book. It's designed to be simple and intuitive yet also deeply transformative. Think of it as an ongoing intimate conversation between your waking and dreaming selves, a dialogue that grows clearer, deeper and more supportive the more frequently you engage with it.

Following this programme will help you move past the confusion and fear that often surround 'bad' dreams and lead you straight to their healing heart. You'll learn to bypass the temptation to overanalyse or panic and instead approach each dream with curiosity, clarity and grounded spiritual insight.

Below is a brief summary of the seven steps. As you read through them, keep in mind that you don't have to do them all instantly and perfectly. Your dreams aren't looking for perfection; they're asking for your presence. If you show up with a genuine desire to better understand your dreams, this method will meet you where you are and take you to where you're ready to go.

In the following pages, we'll explore each step in a little more depth, with real-life dream examples and gentle, empowering practices to help you experience their full potential. For now, let's walk through the structure of your dreamwork toolkit.

Note: Steps One to Four should be done immediately on waking and should take no more than a minute or three. Steps Five to Seven typically take between ten and fifteen minutes and should be done later in the day, ideally just before you fall asleep in the evening.

Step One: the emotion on waking

On waking from a sleep or nap, begin with feeling not with memory. Whether your dream is crystal clear or has been almost entirely forgotten, your first point of contact is always your emotional state upon waking.

Before moving, sitting up, reaching for your phone or beginning your day, pause. Notice how you feel. Are you anxious, sad, confused, relieved, heavy, inspired or numb? Maybe you remember the dream but feel detached from it emotionally. Maybe you don't remember anything, yet you woke up feeling unsettled or elated. Whatever it is, write it down in your dream journal.

This first emotional imprint is your most immediate clue. Dreams are emotional landscapes more than intellectual puzzles and your feeling tone is often the thread that can lead you back into the heart of the dream's message.

Step Two: write down the key symbols

Next, tune into the symbols or images that stand out from the dream and that you think of first. You don't need to capture every detail, just focus on the loudest, most emotionally charged symbols. Choose at least three and no more than five.

These symbols are the dream's language. They may be obvious (a creature, a door, a storm) or more abstract (a colour, a voice, a sensation). Don't worry about interpreting them yet. Just jot them down exactly as they appeared. Don't try to make sense of them.

Step Three: the dream story

Now, give the dream a voice. In a sentence or two, recount the sequence of events as a neutral narrator, using the present tense. Even if you were clearly the main character, try to describe what happened in a more objective, generalized, third-person way so you get into that compassionate, observational role as soon as possible. So, instead of saying, 'I was being chased by monsters,' reframe it as, 'Someone is running away from something threatening.' This step invites a little emotional distance and helps prevent overidentification with the narrative. It allows you to see the dream as a universal story that may carry meaning beyond the personal. Writing the dream out in this way also reveals its story or essence, which often mirrors the structure of a waking-life situation you're currently navigating.

Step Four: name and date your dream

This may seem like a simple or even whimsical step, but it's surprisingly powerful. Giving your dream a title helps crystallize its meaning in your mind. The act of naming helps you form a relationship with the dream, turning it from something confusing or frightening into something familiar and manageable. Writing down the date is important too, as a key part of dream decoding is noticing how your dreams comment on and foreshadow your waking life – and you can't do that cross-referencing without dating your dreams each morning on waking.

Step Five: relate the dream to waking life

Later in the day, ideally before you go to bed so that dreamwork is on your mind when you fall asleep, review your dream journal. Read through the notes you made on waking and zoom in on you. Look at the emotion you wrote down in Step One. Look at the symbols and the dream story. Ask yourself: 'Where in my current waking life does this emotional theme show up? Where am I experiencing similar feelings, patterns or behaviours?' Use free association. What does each symbol remind you of in waking life? What memories, people or feelings does it stir? This spontaneous association begins to reveal the bridge between the dreamworld and your everyday experience. For example, if the dream involves running away, ask yourself honestly: 'What am I running away from in real life?' If the dream shows you lost in a building, reflect: 'Where in my life do I feel directionless or trapped?'

This is where your dream decoding becomes deeply personal and deeply empowering. You are gently beginning to lift the veil between the dreamworld and your waking reality. You're no longer just a witness to the dream; you're an active participant in its healing message.

Step Six: decode with hindsight

Your dreams don't exist in isolation. They are not one-time messages – they are part of an ongoing dialogue between your conscious and unconscious selves. That's why it's so important to look back at your previous dreams and notice patterns, themes and symbolic echoes.

What is being repeated? What emotional themes keep resurfacing? Is there a dream you had weeks or even months ago that connects with this one in some way? Are you noticing that your dreams fall into certain categories?

This hindsight perspective gives you a wider lens. Instead of seeing the current dream as a random message, you begin to see it as a chapter in a much larger soul story that's unfolding over time. That story might be about healing your voice, facing a fear, reclaiming your power or awakening your purpose. But you can't see the bigger picture if you focus only on single dreams. You need the overview.

Often, by returning to earlier dream entries and cross-referencing them with what you've just recorded, you'll uncover a deeper rhythm or spiritual arc in your dreamlife. It's a bit like decoding a map – each dream is a point on the journey.

Step Seven: live the dream

This is the most important step of all. Everything you've uncovered so far – every symbol, every emotion, every insight – is ultimately meant to be applied. Your dreams are not just asking you to understand them; they're asking you to act on them. Reflect on ways you can incorporate their wisdom into your waking life the following day.

This doesn't mean making drastic life changes overnight. It means taking small, soul-aligned actions in your waking life that reflect the messages and guidance your dreams are offering.

If you dream of running from danger, perhaps your waking-life invitation is to stop avoiding a difficult conversation. If you dream of being silenced, maybe it's time to speak your truth in a gentle but firm way. If you dream of drowning, perhaps it's a cue to acknowledge the emotions you've been suppressing and talk to someone about how you feel.

Your dreams are forever trying to move you forward, to help you evolve. And when you begin to live the messages they offer, you start to notice a shift – not just in your dreamlife but in your waking life too. You begin to feel more aligned, more empowered, more in touch with your intuition and inner knowing. You move from being haunted by your dreams to being guided by them.

Seeing Your Dreams Clearly

Once you begin to systematically apply these seven steps – consistently, gently and with an open heart – you'll find that even the most disturbing dreams begin to lose their grip. They will no longer feel like something to dread or suppress but something to work with, learn from and grow through.

Remember, your dreams are not problems. They are honest and non-judgemental mirrors. And now that you have a method that allows you to see clearly what they are trying to show you, it's time to explore each of these seven steps in greater depth. The real-life dream examples and practical tools below will help you learn how to apply the steps to a variety of situations and bring the process to life. You'll discover how easy it is to access the wisdom of your inner dream therapist and how transformational that relationship can be. Let's go.

Step One: The Emotion on Waking

The very first and often most revealing clue to decoding a dream is how you feel when you wake up. Not what you remember. Not what happened. But how you feel, in your body, in your breath, in your mind and in your heart.

This step is deceptively simple and easy to do, so don't overlook its power. Dreams speak through emotion far more than they do through logic or linear storylines. Even if the dream itself quickly fades, the emotional residue often lingers – an anxious flutter in your chest, a sense of dread, a rush of joy, a heavy weight in your limbs. This emotional signature is your soul's first attempt to get your attention.

Think of this emotional tone as the energetic 'envelope' your dream arrives in. Before you open it, before you analyse or interpret your dream, just notice what it's wrapped in. That feeling is your direct line to what your inner self is trying to express.

Why emotion matters so much

Your dreaming mind doesn't waste time sugar-coating. It shows you, without filters, what you're feeling beneath the surface. The emotion you wake up with often bypasses the rational mind and speaks straight from the subconscious. For example:

- If you wake up feeling panicked, even from a dream you barely remember, the chances are something in waking life is triggering anxiety or avoidance.
- If you feel peaceful after a vivid dream of visiting someone who has passed, the dream may be a soul-level reassurance or emotional closure.
- If you're angry but the dream seemed uneventful, your anger may be buried; not expressed in waking life but safely released in the dream.

Sometimes the emotion is the dream's whole message. Other times, it points you to what the dream's story is asking you to face. Either way, recording the feeling is essential. It sets the emotional tone that the rest of your decoding will build upon.

What if there's no emotion?

Occasionally, you'll recall a dream with surprising clarity but feel emotionally flat or detached. The dream might feel like watching a movie or a memory projected on a screen, rather than something you lived through.

When this happens, it's worth noting. Emotionally neutral dreams aren't necessarily meaningless; they often belong in a different category altogether. These 'projector-like' dreams may fall under the literal or psychic/foreshadowing categories covered in Chapter Six. In such cases, the absence of emotion can be a clue that the dream is delivering information rather than emotional processing.

That's why this first step of simply naming how you feel is so vital. It immediately begins to sort your dreams into emotional versus informational, symbolic versus literal.

A practice: anchor the emotion

Upon waking, before you move, speak or reach for your phone, try this gentle awareness practice:

1. Stay still. Keep your eyes closed and your body relaxed. Notice whatever thoughts, words, associations, images or symbols come to mind.

2. Scan your body with feelings of love. Begin at your toes and slowly move your attention upward. Do you feel any tightness, heaviness, warmth or tingling? Are certain areas relaxed or tense? Especially take note of the most highly intuitive centres of your body, your heart and your gut, which may well hold dream memories and feelings.
3. Name the feeling. Without judging or trying to understand it, simply name the dominant emotion. Is it fear? Sadness? Curiosity? Relief? Confusion?
4. Breathe into it. Take a few slow breaths into the part of your body that holds the strongest sensation. Allow the emotion to be there, even for just a moment.
5. Write one sentence in your dream journal. Note down the emotional state and any physical sensations, even if the dream content is vague or missing.

The simple act of tuning into your body and your mind with inquisitiveness and care on waking, even for only one or two minutes, creates a clear and conscious connection between your dreamlife and your waking awareness. Over time, you'll notice patterns in your emotional landscape and your dreams will start to feel less chaotic and more purposeful. Remember: your feelings are the thread that connects your sleeping world to your waking one. Follow that thread and it will always lead you towards insight.

Rather than reaching for your phone on waking, focus on your inner world. This can be life changing. What you do first thing is like putting the key in the ignition of a car: it sets the tone for the day ahead. If you automatically reach for your phone first thing, you are directing your attention to the material world and all its busy demands and setting the tone of 'outside in'. Instead, stay still a while and look within, setting an empowered tone for the rest of the day.

Step Two: Symbols – Your Soul's Secret Language

After identifying how you felt upon waking, your next step in decoding a dream is to focus on the key symbols that stood out. Emotions and symbols are the language your dreams use to communicate with you – they are the poetic metaphors of your soul, shaped by your own life experiences, beliefs and subconscious mind.

Dreams rarely speak to us directly. Instead, they wrap their messages in images, actions and strange juxtapositions that often seem nonsensical until we begin to unpack them. This symbolic language may be unfamiliar at first, but once you start listening and learning how it speaks, you'll find that it's incredibly rich, wise and deeply personal.

Why you must keep it simple

One of the most common mistakes people make when working with their dreams is trying to capture everything. Every single detail, every strange occurrence, every background object.

But dreams are like abstract paintings – overanalysing every brushstroke can drown out the overall message.

To avoid this kind of dream overcrowding and to save yourself time when writing down your dreams in the morning, focus on no more than three to five key symbols. These should be the ones that stand out to you most – the symbols that linger, echo or strike an emotional chord, even if you don't know why. They are at the top of your mental inbox for a reason.

For example:

- You dreamed you were lost in a forest and there were loads of strange animals and plants, but what sticks with you most is not so much the forest and the trees and plants but the image of a locked wooden door in the middle of a path.
- You dreamed of being back at school and there were so many things going on there, but the thing you can't shake is the repeating sound of a school bell.
- You dreamed of flying and of all the things you saw it is the image of a black bird following close behind that haunts you.

These symbols are your dream's shorthand. They condense complex emotions and experiences into a single potent image. Instead of overwhelming you with explanations, your psyche delivers insight through visual metaphor. That's why it's important to let your symbols choose you, not the other way around.

Dreams speak in emotion and symbol

Emotion (Step One) is the tone. Symbol is the translation. Your dream uses both in tandem. The emotional signature shows how something feels; the symbol shows what it's about. Together, they create a two-part message from your unconscious mind that encourages you to ask questions.

Imagine dreaming of a crumbling house. That's the symbol. You wake up feeling anxious and sad and that's the emotional tone. When you bring those two together, the dream might be highlighting fears about instability, loss or transition, especially if your waking life includes major change, like a house move or relationship upheaval.

Or consider a dream where you're holding a newborn baby. The feeling on waking is excitement and awe but also terror, because you aren't sure if the baby is yours. Perhaps the baby doesn't represent a literal child but rather a new beginning – a project, relationship or version of yourself that's just coming into being and of which you have yet to achieve mastery.

symbol + emotion = questions that can bring insight

Like great poetry, art and music, dreams aren't here to hand you clear-cut answers. Instead, they invite you to feel and to ask better, deeper questions – questions that can lead to wiser choices in your waking life. The real power of dreams lies not in solving problems but in sparking your fascination. It's the not knowing that activates your mind, pushing you to explore, experiment and discover. While answers can bring a sense of finality, questions keep you moving forward, learning and evolving – and evolving is the meaning of life. The more comfortable you become with uncertainty as a positive force for personal and spiritual growth, the more you'll gain from your dreamwork. Growth begins where certainty ends and doubt steps in.

A practice: dream-symbol recall

1. Remain still upon waking. Once you have identified the emotion (Step One), remain still in bed with your eyes closed. Take the focus away from emotion now and ask yourself softly: 'What did I see/feel in the dream?' Focus on visuals, words and symbols only: objects, creatures, landscapes, strange items or repeating imagery.
2. Write down two to five symbols in your dream diary. Write only the symbols that stand out. Use simple words or short phrases, such as 'red door' or 'glass box' or 'black bird'. There's no need to describe or interpret what happened – just capture what was there.

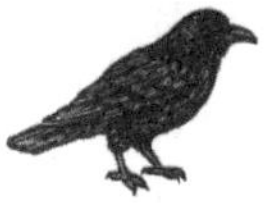

3. Repeat this process every morning upon waking, listing two to five standout dream symbols.

When you give attention to your dream's key symbols and approach them with curiosity instead of control, the deeper meaning begins to emerge. You'll start to notice patterns, recurring images and inner metaphors that build over time. These symbols are like spiritual breadcrumbs, encouraging you to brainstorm and ask questions, leading you towards growth, truth and healing.

So, as you move through your dream journal, pause after each dream. Ask yourself: 'What are the loudest images here? What won't leave me alone? What am I drawn to, even if it makes no sense?' Write them down. Trust the process. Your soul is speaking to you like a poet in the language of symbols and now you're learning how to remember and listen. Indeed, a dream-decoding hack is to think of every dream as a poem all about you. Interpret it in the same way, looking beneath the surface for meaning as you would when interpreting a poem.

Step Three: The Dream Story – Seeing it Like a Storyteller, not a Character

Now that you've identified the emotion (Step One) and the symbols (Step Two), it's time to bring the dream into focus as a whole experience – a story. But there's a very specific and transformative way to do this. You're going to write the dream in the present tense, to remind you that your dreams always comment on what is currently going on in your waking life; and, most importantly, you are going to approach your dreams from a neutral, objective point of view.

Instead of retelling the dream as something that happened to you, you'll describe it as if you're watching a scene unfold – a scene that could be happening to anyone. This shift in perspective may feel unusual at first, but it's key to accessing the deeper meaning.

Why objectivity matters

When you write your dream using 'I' statements – 'I'm running', 'I'm trapped', 'I'm screaming' – you lock yourself into the emotional drama of the dream. Emotions are vital, and you have already explored them in Step One, but staying inside the dream as a character can cloud your ability to see the bigger picture.

By stepping outside the dream and describing it generically – 'Someone is running', 'A person is trapped' – you begin to view it like a film director or storyteller. You become the observer rather than the actor. This subtle shift creates emotional space and gives your intuitive mind room to work. You're no longer stuck in the feeling; you're witnessing the pattern.

When you observe a dream from the outside, you see it as a message, not a meltdown. Let's look at the difference between personal and objective perspectives using a couple of examples:

> Personal: 'I'm on a train that's speeding out of control and no one is driving it. I try to stop it, but the brakes don't work. I'm terrified.'

> Objective: 'Someone is on a fast-moving train with no conductor. They try to stop the train, but the brakes fail. Panic sets in.'

Without the personal pronoun, you can more easily step back and ask: 'What does this image say about loss of control? Who or what in my life feels like it's running too fast with no direction?' You're now watching the symbolic structure of the dream unfold, not just reliving your fear. It puts you in the driving seat.

> Personal: 'I'm trying to call my partner, but the phone won't dial. I get more and more frustrated.'

> Objective: 'A person is trying to connect with someone important, but communication is blocked. Frustration builds.'

Suddenly, the dream becomes a universal theme – communication breakdown, emotional disconnection – that you can explore with greater clarity.

A practice: step outside the dream

Here's a simple exercise to help you shift into that neutral dream-narrator role:

1. Close your eyes and revisit the dream scene in your mind, as if you're watching it on a screen.
2. Imagine you are not the character but the observer, like someone watching a short film.
3. Ask yourself: 'What is the main character trying to do? What is preventing them from doing it? How does the "film" make me feel as a viewer?'
4. Now, write the dream out in the present tense, without using personal pronouns. Replace 'I' with 'someone' or 'a person'. Limit your description to no more than one or two sentences outlining the core actions, feelings and setting of the dream.

You might be surprised how powerful this observational shift from first to third person can be. It allows patterns and metaphors to emerge that you couldn't see when you were emotionally entangled in the dream.

The power of perspective

This step isn't about detachment or denial. While Step One allows you to honour the emotional weight of your dream, Step Three is about giving yourself the gift of perspective. Objectivity doesn't mean distance; it means clarity. It allows the message behind the emotion to rise to the surface.

When you learn to describe your dream story like an outsider looking in, you invite your inner wisdom to step forward. You shift from being overwhelmed to being empowered. You begin to see the narrative arc, not just the chaos.

And when you can observe your dreams this way, you'll start to observe your waking life differently too, with more insight, more compassion and more awareness of the stories you're unconsciously living. Remember: your dreams are telling stories and your job is to know how to listen.

Step Four: Name and Date Your Dream – Let it Tell You What it Is

Once you've uncovered the emotion, decoded the symbols and described the dream story, you will be ready for a creative and intuitive moment in your dreamwork: giving your dream a name.

This may seem like a small step but it's powerful. Naming your dream helps to distil its meaning into a single phrase or image that lingers in your mind. It transforms the dream from a chaotic blur into something you can hold, revisit and understand over time. It's like creating a label on a spiritual message from your subconscious. When you name a dream, you claim it and begin to see where it fits in the greater conversation your mind is having with you. Don't overthink this step; just go with whatever immediately comes to you.

And then make sure you put a date beside the name of your dream, because the only way to see how your dreams comment on or foreshadow your waking life is to have that date in place. Indeed, you might want to keep your dream journal side by side with your waking journal, if you keep one – perhaps use one side of the page for your daily schedule and the other side of the page for your dream recall. Over time you will start to see how your dreams act like a poetic voiceover commenting on your waking life.

Why naming the dream matters

Giving your dream a title acts like sealing a letter from the subconscious. It's a way of honouring the message and taking it seriously. A name gives the dream definition; it turns something ephemeral into something memorable. As with the previous step, try to keep that all-important observational approach when deciding on a title.

You might call a dream:

- 'The Crumbling Bridge'
- 'No One Can Hear Them'
- 'The House with No Doors'
- 'The Golden Light'
- 'The Message from the Stranger'

Choose a name that captures the essence, image or emotional truth of the dream. It doesn't need to be clever or profound, just honest. This small creative act brings clarity and clarity brings healing. And if you are stuck, you can simply name it after the most striking symbol from your list.

A practice: title and time

Try this reflective exercise after recording the emotional tone, symbols and story in your dream journal:

1. Close your eyes, take a breath and ask: 'If this dream were a book or film, what would its title be?' Avoid personal pronouns such as 'I' or 'Me' in your title. Focus on the bigger picture.
2. Write it down immediately without overthinking.
3. If you had several dream stories, do the same for each one. It is rare to wake up with just one dream memory on your mind as you do dream several times a night, every night.
4. Make sure you record the date of your dream.
5. Your waking dreamwork is now done. The morning is a busy time and your to-do list for the day ahead is calling your attention. Attend to it, safe in the knowledge that you have recorded the essential details of your dream and will return to it later in the day to begin the real business of decoding.

Why this step deepens everything

When you give your dream a name and date, you create a spiritual snapshot in time. You begin to see how this dream fits into the greater mosaic of your inner life and prepares you to begin a dialogue with it.

Next, we'll explore how your dreams work as a series, not in isolation, and how hindsight often reveals meanings that weren't obvious at first. You need time away from your dream first, though and should come back to the process once the day's busyness and distractions are over.

For now, take a moment to honour the dream on your mind. Title it. Date it. Let it take its place in the sacred library of your unconscious, where healing and understanding are always unfolding, ready to reveal its secrets when you are ready.

Step Five: Relate the Dream to Waking Life – Finding the Mirror

Steps Five, Six and Seven should be performed several hours after recalling your dream, ideally before sleeping. Your brain is very impressionable at this time, so if you are thinking about the messages of your dreams then you will likely wake up the next morning with even clearer dream recall.

Find your dream journal and read through the notes you made on waking that morning. You should have the emotional tone, some symbols, a dream story, title and date.

Now it is time to take the most vital step of all – relating your dream to your waking life.

This is the moment where the mystery starts to dissolve and meaning emerges. Without this step, dreams remain strange little stories floating in the dark. But once you ask how the dream connects to your lived experience, it becomes a mirror that reflects parts of your life you may not have fully seen or acknowledged.

Your dream is always about you

Regardless of how surreal or nonsensical the dream may seem, it's about you – more specifically, it's about where you are emotionally, mentally or spiritually at the time of dreaming. Every symbol, sensation, story, image, sound and so on in your dream is a metaphor for some aspect of your current mindset or a situation in your waking life. Remember, everything in your dreamwork is about YOU.

That's why your personal response to dream symbols or themes takes priority over online or book-form dream decoders, which can offer only the common or universal interpretations. Go to those resources only if your personal association yields nothing and you want help to kickstart your symbolic thinking. To illustrate this point, I always offer the example of a dream about dogs. If you love dogs, the association is a positive one – and you will find that positive association in dream dictionaries you consult; but if you feel anxious around dogs, your interpretation of a dog cameoing in your dreamworld will be the opposite.

In short, trust your own immediate response first and if nothing specific breaks through into your awareness then by all means read generic interpretations to see if anything resonates. Indeed, I often recommend going through all the interpretations until you get an 'aha' moment, because the chances are that whatever prompted it will be the correct meaning and one that surprises, inspires or uplifts you. A dream interpretation that drags you down or feels predictable is always incorrect, because dreams are your intuition talking to you and your intuition is always on your side. It's also fine if nothing stands out – just keep pondering the dream meaning. Meanings sometimes take days or even years to surface. Sometimes they never surface at all. Trust that your dreaming mind is doing the undercover work and that it knows what it is doing, because it does.

The language of dreams might be bizarre but their purpose is very practical. Remind yourself that your dreams are offering you a way to process what you're struggling with, integrate what you're avoiding, illuminate what you've been ignoring or they foreshadow the potential future your current mindset is attracting. Every dream is trying to draw your attention to something real happening inside you. Now is your time to find out what that something is.

The process of linking the dreamworld to your real world takes honesty, courage and a little practice but it also brings the most reward. Ask yourself: 'Where is this same feeling, dynamic or behaviour showing up in my waking life?'

By way of example, let's say you dreamed:

A person is trapped inside a small room with no windows. They scream but no one hears.

You woke up feeling anxious and isolated. You noted the symbol of the windowless room and the inability to be heard. Now ask: 'Where in my life do I feel emotionally trapped or unseen?'

Perhaps you're in a relationship or job where your voice feels silenced. Maybe there's something you've been keeping inside, afraid to express. The dream is holding up a mirror to that and letting you know that for your own wellbeing you need to find ways around that.

Or imagine you dreamed:

Someone is carrying a child up a mountain. The path is steep and they feel exhausted, but they keep going.

You woke feeling both heavy and determined. One symbol is the child; another is the climb. Now ask: 'What responsibility am I carrying that feels overwhelming but necessary?'

Maybe you're caring for a loved one or nurturing a creative project. The dream may be reminding you of your strength, while also gently acknowledging your fatigue and need for self-care. The dream doesn't give you answers; it gives you the right questions.

A practice: the dream-to-life bridge and free association

To deepen this step, try this simple reflection practice and free-association technique after reading your dream:

1. Review the emotional tone, symbols and story you have written down.
2. Ask: 'Where do I feel this emotion in my waking life right now? What or who does this symbol remind me of? What situation does this dream seem to echo?'
3. Use the following sentence starter to guide you: 'This dream might be about my feelings around . . .' Let it be a guess. You don't need certainty, just a willingness to connect the dots. If nothing comes to you right away, trust that the connection will surface later. Often, just asking the question opens the space for clarity to arrive when you are ready for it.
4. Now take a deep breath and practise one of the most effective dream-analysis tools available: free association. Think in the language of similes, symbols and metaphors and interpret your dream as if it were a poem. Many poems don't make complete sense on first reading. You need to look beneath the literal meaning of the words to decipher the real meaning. Choose one

symbol – for example, 'black bird'. Then, in your journal, quickly jot down the first thoughts, memories, ideas or images it brings up for you – perhaps 'black bird → omen, mystery, death, intelligence, messages, freedom'. Keep it spontaneous. Don't try to make sense of it or censor your responses. The key is to bypass your logical mind and let your intuition speak freely.

What you're doing here is bridging your personal associations to the dream's symbols. This is important because while some dream imagery is collective (for instance, water often symbolizes emotion), much of it is highly personal. A snake may mean fear and danger to one person but transformation and healing to another, depending on life experience, cultural background or even childhood memories. By free associating, you're letting your inner self tell you what the symbol means and how it relates to your waking life, not relying on external definitions or dream dictionaries. You're decoding the dream in the language of your own soul.

Free association is so powerful because it cuts through the noise. It stops you from overthinking and helps you connect instinctively to the wisdom within. It also opens doors to surprising insights about your waking life. You may think a symbol is meaningless, only to discover it echoes something buried deep in your heart.

The dream as a wakeup call

This step is not about intellectualizing or overanalysing. It's about feeling into the meaning of your night vision. Your dreams are always offering feedback on how aligned or misaligned you are with your values, boundaries or emotional truth.

Sometimes the connection is obvious, but Step Five often provides a surprising and energizing new perspective. At other times, it reveals something you aren't ready to admit. But it's always compassionate. Your dreaming mind isn't here to criticize; it's trying to give you an honest reflection to help you course correct, to bring unconscious emotion into conscious awareness so you can proceed with greater self-understanding and self-kindness. Indeed, the mark of a well-decoded dream is its ability to energize and empower you. It is worth repeating, because this is so crucial, that any dream interpretation that drains or diminishes you is the wrong interpretation.

When you take the time to explore what your dream reflects about your waking life, your inner world and outer world begin to harmonize. Your dream no longer feels random or overwhelming; it feels like a message from your deeper self, inviting you to seize the moment and grow.

Step Six: Hindsight – Seeing the Pattern Behind the Pieces

Dreams are rarely one-off events. They are not isolated messages dropped randomly into the night. Instead, they are more like chapters in an ongoing story of interwoven messages from your inner world, stitched together by time, memory and emotion. In other words, your dreams often follow a narrative thread, with each dream continuing the story of amazing you.

This is why Step Six asks you to engage with one of the most neglected but most important dream-decoding stages: looking back at your dreams from the previous few days.

Hindsight turns confusion into clarity. It helps you see connections that weren't obvious in the moment and reveals the longer arc of emotional and spiritual growth your dreams are gently guiding you through. It also shows you how your dreams are always commentating on your waking life – like a poetic voiceover – and how they can often foreshadow what is to come.

This step asks you to go back through your dream journal, not to re-analyse or obsess but simply to observe and notice patterns. When you look at your dreams in sequence, you begin to see how they work in layers. Themes repeat. Symbols evolve. Emotions shift. Patterns surface. Meanings flow. And the same soul-level concerns arise repeatedly until you're ready to face them, heal them or integrate them.

Dreams speak in series

Just like a TV series or a novel, your dreams have recurring characters, plotlines and motifs. A symbol that felt random in one dream might reappear in another dream or nightmare weeks later and suddenly take on meaning. An emotion that overwhelmed you once might feel softer now, because something inside you has shifted.

Let's say that on three nights in one month you dream about being lost in a city. The setting is different each time but the feeling is the same: disorientation, urgency, confusion. Only when you review your dreams in hindsight do you realize that they all occurred during a time of career change or personal uncertainty. The repetition is your inner self trying to help you navigate this change and accept the uncertainty.

Or perhaps you dreamed about a black dog months ago and thought nothing of it. Now it's reappeared in a new dream – this time guiding you to safety. Hindsight reveals that the dog represents an inner strength or guardian energy you've slowly come to trust.

These patterns are subtle but powerful. They show that your psyche is not random but intelligent, compassionate and constantly invested in your growth.

The never-ending and constantly evolving timeline

One of the most beautiful discoveries you'll make through hindsight is how your emotional tone changes over time. When you look back at previous dreams, you might notice that nightmares become less intense. Symbols of struggle turn into symbols of resolution. Dreams that once felt threatening now feel empowering. Different nightmare symbols emerge.

These shifts often happen so gradually that you don't notice them day by day, but in hindsight they're undeniable. It's like watching yourself learn, grow and heal in slow motion – and that is incredibly validating. You may also start noticing patterns and that your dreams fall into certain categories, such as those listed below. This is when things really become interesting.

1. **Cathartic dreams.** These dreams exist to release stored emotion. They may feel dramatic or chaotic, but over time their purpose is emotional cleansing. You might dream of crying, shouting, falling or extreme frustration. You wake up feeling lighter, even if the dream was difficult.
2. **Confrontational dreams.** These dreams bring you face to face with fears, avoidance or inner conflict. You may be chased, judged, trapped or in conflict with someone you know. They ask: 'What are you not facing in real life?'
3. **Recurring dreams.** These dreams repeat over time, often with slight variations. Recurring dreams usually signal a persistent issue that hasn't been resolved or acknowledged. They are your psyche's version of a gentle (or not-so-gentle) nudge to learn a lesson not yet learned or to better understand something about yourself.

4. **Problem-solving dreams.** These dreams offer insight, solutions or clarity about a specific situation or dilemma. They can feel more structured or even strangely logical. You may wake up with a new highly creative idea, a resolution or a sudden knowing.
5. **Integration dreams.** These dreams show internal healing or personal growth in progress. You might dream of reconciling with someone, finding a lost object or stepping through a door. These dreams are often quieter but carry a sense of emotional peace or spiritual resolution.
6. **Psychic dreams.** These dreams are telepathic or offer a connection to the afterlife. For example, they may be visions of departed loved ones or dreams that are precognitive in that they predict future events, situations or mindsets when you experience a moment of déjà rêvé ('already dreamed') – a sense that you have already dreamed about something that is now playing out in your waking life. Psychic dreams can feel emotionally neutral or strangely vivid and often 'play out like a movie'. If you wake with strong recall but little emotion, the dream may fall into this category. These dreams are less about your inner world and more about your psychic and spiritual awakening. They can and do occur – and more often than we are led to believe. We will discuss psychic dreams in more detail in Chapter Six.

7. **Literal warnings.** Dreams that can be interpreted literally are rare but it is always worth ruling out the potential for literal meaning. For example, if you dreamed that your teeth were falling out, do you need to book a checkup with your dentist? Usually, such dreams are symbolic and metaphorical, but it's only with the benefit of hindsight that you will know whether a dream was truly a literal warning. (More about how to identify and work with those literal and psychic dreams in Chapter Six.)

A practice: dream-reflection session

Try this practice once a week or at the end of a significant life period:

1. Set aside at least 15 minutes with your dream journal.
2. Reread the dreams you've recorded from the past few weeks or months.
3. As you read, look for: repeated symbols or settings; recurring emotions or themes; and any signs of progression, such as dreams becoming lighter, more resolved or less fearful – though take note if the opposite is true too and you notice your dreams becoming more intense or darker.
4. Make a short summary list. For example, 'Three dreams about water, each with different emotional

tone', 'Recurring dream of being unable to speak', 'Shift from being chased to finally stopping and turning around'.

5. Reflect with compassion. Ask: 'What is my soul trying to teach me over time? What changes are my dreams reflecting to me?' You might even give each week a 'dream theme', like a chapter title in the book of your inner life.
6. See if you can put some of your dreams into any of the following categories:
    - **Cathartic** dreams that allow you to release repressed emotion or trauma
    - **Confrontational** dreams that challenge you to face fears or truths you've been avoiding
    - **Recurring** dreams that repeat until their message is understood or integrated
    - **Problem-solving** dreams that offer creative insight or clarity around a specific issue
    - **Integration** dreams with themes of personal and spiritual growth
    - **Psychic** dreams that may carry intuitive glimpses of future possibilities or collective themes

Gently place a dream into one of the six categories, trusting your first instinct. Now ask: 'What is this dream trying to do? Is it clearing, confronting, solving, repeating, predicting or healing?'

If it feels like it fits into more than one category, that's fine – many dreams blend categories. Perhaps you can create an entirely new category of your own. The point is to begin thinking of your dream as a type of message, which helps you understand why you had that dream, why it came, what it wants from you and what kind of action or inner reflection it might be pointing towards.

Maybe this is your third cathartic dream in a row. Or your recurring nightmare is finally shifting towards resolution. Or maybe you've had your first psychic-style dream and are starting to open to intuitive messages from beyond your own story. Whatever the case, this step helps you track the themes and patterns of your dreamworld and that dream detective work gives insight, direction and the beautiful feeling of being in dialogue with your own soul.

The gift of looking back

Dreams exist outside of time and are often way ahead of us. They look back at us and help us sense what's coming before we consciously know. This is why hindsight can feel like a revelation – because suddenly a dream from weeks or months ago makes perfect sense considering what's happening right now.

Looking back on your dreams also builds trust in your inner wisdom or intuition. You'll begin to realize you've always known, deep down. Your dreams were showing you, even when you couldn't yet see it in your waking life.

This step doesn't require expertise; it simply asks for attention. When you lovingly review your dreams as an ongoing series, you begin to see that nothing is wasted. Every symbol, every emotion, every strange and beautiful scene is part of a larger dialogue between your conscious self and your soul. You also understand that your dreams don't want a one-night stand. They want a long-term committed and loving relationship with you. Don't become obsessed with one particularly memorable dream. See it as part of the longest-running and most spectacular show you will ever watch – the never-ending story of amazing YOU.

The dreamworld is layered, cyclical and wise beyond measure. Hindsight lets you witness its unfolding. From this place of ongoing reflection, you're ready to take the final, most important step: bringing your dream wisdom into your waking life.

Step Seven: Live the Dream – Turning Insight into Action

After moving through the first six steps – tuning into your waking emotion, decoding symbols, writing the story, claiming the dream, making the connection to your life and looking back with hindsight – there's only one thing left for you to do: live the dream.

This is where your dreamwork becomes real. It's not just

something you journal about or reflect upon inside your head; it's something you embody. Your dream has given you a message, a mirror, a metaphor. Now it's time to bring that message into your waking world and let it shape how you live, love, speak and grow. Dreams are only as powerful as the positive actions they inspire in your waking life once you understand them.

Dreamwork is soul work

At their heart, dreams are not just stories; they're invitations to engage in personal and spiritual growth. Every single one asks you to evolve. Sometimes that evolution is subtle: a shift in perspective, a deeper compassion, a small truth you finally admit to yourself. Sometimes it's bigger: a decision you've been avoiding, a boundary you need to set, a relationship you need to heal or move away from. No matter the size, the invitation to change your life for the better is always there.

- A dream about being lost in a storm may be inviting you to slow down and find inner direction.
- A dream about speaking on a stage might be nudging you to express your truth.
- A dream about running from a shadow may be asking you to stop and face a part of yourself with love, not fear.

If you understand the message but never apply it, the dream remains theoretical and stuck in your head. But taking even one small action to honour the dream allows the dream to enter your body and your life and this is where real transformation begins.

Small shifts, big meaning

You don't need to make grand gestures to 'live the dream'. Often, it's the smallest, most intentional actions that have the greatest impact. Here are a few gentle ways you might integrate a dream's message:

- If your dream was about feeling voiceless, speak up in a conversation where you'd usually stay silent.
- If your dream showed you stuck in a place with no exits, take one small step to move forward in a stagnant area of your life.
- If your dream featured a symbol of freedom, like flying, give yourself a day of unstructured time or permission to pursue a joy you've been denying.
- If your dream showed violent confrontation, have an honest check-in with yourself or someone close to you.
- If your dream held a healing image, bring that energy into your day with a meditation, journal prompt or physical gesture such as going for a mindful walk.

What matters most is alignment. Any action, no matter how simple, that reflects the inner truth revealed by your dream is a form of spiritual integration.

A practice: breathing life into your dream

After decoding a dream:

1. Ask yourself: 'What is this dream asking me to pay attention to?'
2. Then ask: 'What would change if I truly lived by the message of this dream today?'
3. Lastly, ask: 'What is one small action I can take to honour the insight I received?' Write that action down and if possible perform the action before the day ends. Don't wait for the right moment, because it won't come; start now with your noble intention.
4. Choose one symbol that is safe in your dream. The next day, bring that symbol into your waking awareness to show your dreaming mind you are listening and taking its precious wisdom seriously and to heart. For example, if your dream featured roses, buy yourself a bunch; and when you have that symbol in your hands, honour the sacred connection you are consciously creating as the bridge it is between your waking and your dreaming life. Even symbolic actions can create deep inner shifts. For instance, if your dream involved a closed door, you might literally open a window or door while repeating the affirmation: 'I am ready for new beginnings.' These small rituals send powerful signals to your subconscious that you are listening and responding.

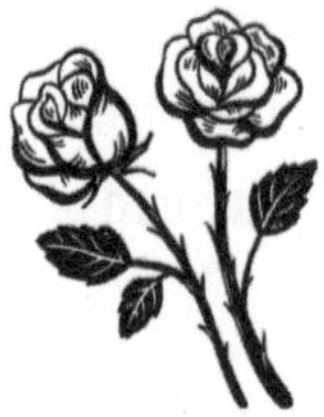

The wisdom was always within you

When you proactively live the wisdom of your dream, you affirm something essential: that your inner world is not separate from your outer life. That your soul speaks not just through signs and synchronicities but through your very own imagination and intuition. That your dreams are not just nighttime stories but sacred blueprints for healing, change and self-realization.

This final step is all about the power of daily practice. Walking the dream talk. Keep returning to your dreams. Keep listening. Keep living what they're teaching you. Some mornings the message will be loud and clear. Other times it will whisper and unfold slowly. Trust both. Because when you begin to live your dreams, you're not just decoding your sleep – you're waking up to who you truly are. And that is the real magic of dreamwork.

Now that you've learned the seven steps, you have a toolkit for navigating even the most intense or extreme dreams. Later in the book, we'll further explore how to tell the difference between personal dreams and that rarer kind of dreams that may be literal or psychic in nature. Because sometimes, your dream isn't just about you it's about something far bigger. For now, though, the nightlight stays firmly on you.

A Terrifying Dream, Transformed: The Seven Steps in Action

Let's bring the seven steps together by walking through an example – something raw, unsettling and deeply emotional. This is a dream many people have had in some form or another. Although it seems at first glance to be purely nightmarish, when it is decoded it reveals something much more profound.

> The dreamer is in a house. They don't recognize it, but it feels like theirs. The walls are old, the rooms cramped. Suddenly, flames burst out from under the floorboards. The fire spreads too quickly. The dreamer tries to run, but the doors are stuck. Smoke fills the air. They scream, but no one hears. They wake up in a panic, heart racing.

Step One: Emotion on Waking

The dreamer writes: 'I woke up terrified. My chest felt tight. It stayed with me all morning and I couldn't shake the fear.' This emotional residue is the most important clue – fear, suffocation and helplessness are trying to surface from somewhere within the waking self.

Step Two: Key Symbols

The dreamer notes three main symbols: burning house, stuck doors, no one hears them.

Step Three: Dream Story

The dream is rewritten objectively: 'A person is inside a house that suddenly catches fire. They try to escape, but the exits are blocked. They call out for help, but no one responds. Panic grows.'

Step Four: Name and Date It

The dreamer names the dream 'No Way Out' and writes down the date on which it was dreamed.

Step Five: Link to Waking Life

The dreamer reflects: 'I've been feeling overwhelmed at work and in my relationship. Like everything's closing in and I can't find a way out. I've kept a lot inside, anger, frustration, fear. I've also felt like no one is really listening when I try to talk about it.'

The dream is now clearly mirroring the dreamer's emotional reality: burnout, emotional isolation and the pressure of responsibilities building to a breaking point. The dreamer uses free association to reflect on the three main symbols and apply them to their waking life: burning house = chaos, destruction, home life falling apart; stuck doors = no way out, trapped, powerless; no one hears = I feel invisible, abandoned, ignored.

Step Six: Hindsight

Looking back through their dream journal, the dreamer notices a pattern, with previous dreams including themes of being chased, trapped or silenced. This one feels like an emotional climax. It may be the psyche's final push: 'Deal with this now.'

There's also a progression, from external threats in earlier dreams to now being trapped within a burning 'home', suggesting that the inner self is crying out for attention. After more reflection, the dreamer decides it's a confrontational and cathartic dream. It's forcing them to face the emotional fire they've been suppressing and perhaps allowing that release to happen before it consumes more of their peace.

Step Seven: Live the Dream

The dreamer decides to act. They schedule a therapy session they've been putting off. They also have a long-overdue conversation with their partner and begin to explore stress-reducing practices. Symbolically, they light a candle in the evening, not to mimic the dream's destruction but to honour the fire as a symbol of transformation. A fire can destroy, yes, but it also clears space for something new to grow.

This dream, alarming as it was, became a turning point. Not because it was 'just a dream' but because it was the dreamer's truth, spoken in the poetic, emotionally charged language of the unconscious.

Dreaming down the moon

There is some intriguing research suggesting that the phases of the moon may influence dreaming, mood and sleep. For example, one study found that around a full moon participants experienced shorter periods of deep sleep and took longer to fall asleep (with about 20 minutes less sleep and a 30 per cent drop in delta-wave activity) under controlled laboratory conditions.*

In practice, this could mean that nights when the moon is full (and thus the night sky is more illuminated) lead to lighter sleep. For some people, this could in turn increase the likelihood of vivid dreams or even nightmares, because awakenings or arousals are more frequent and the boundary between REM (dream) sleep and wakefulness is more fragile. Meanwhile, some dreamworkers and anecdotal accounts suggest a shift towards more creative, reflective or even precognitive dreaming during the waning-moon

* Christian Cajochen et al., 'Evidence that the Lunar Cycle Influences Human Sleep', *Current Biology*, 23(15) (2013), pp. 1,485–8, doi: 10.1016/j.cub.2013.06.029.

phase (after full moon, as the lunar illumination decreases). This is possibly because the diminished 'stimulus' of moonlight contributes to reduced environmental arousal, permitting deeper access to the subconscious.

One of the researchers who links dreaming, precognition and subtle cycles is my *Premonition Code* co-author, the neuroscientist Julia Mossbridge. In her review of the precognition evidence and theory,* she describes how dreams may function as a window into future-oriented processing. She also notes that her post-hoc analysis of online trials showed peaks in participation and higher accuracy during the last-quarter/waning-crescent lunar phases compared to the full/waning-gibbous phases, though this is preliminary and not yet widely replicated.

In summary: nights around full moon may invite lighter, more fragmented sleep (potentially increasing the risk of nightmares) because of increased nocturnal illumination and arousal, while the waning-moon period may offer a more conducive backdrop to deeper, creative or even precognitive dream states.

* Julia Mossbridge, 'Precognition at the Boundaries: An Empirical Review and Theoretical Discussion', *Journal of Anomalous Experience and Cognition*, 3(1) (2023), pp. 5–41, doi: 10.31156/jaex.24216.

From Nightmare to Nightlight

When you learn to decode dreams in this way, you begin to see that every dream is an opportunity for personal growth. Even your darkest dreams and nightmares are not punishments or predictions; they are not your enemy. They are unfiltered glimpses of your deepest truths.

And for a variety of reasons some of those truths live deep in the shadow self, the parts of yourself you've denied, repressed or disowned in your waking. That's what we'll explore in the next chapter. Because if you're ready to truly transform, to reclaim every part of yourself and to face your fear not as an enemy but as a teacher, then shadow work is the next crucial step on your extreme-dreaming journey. Often, intensely menacing dreams or nightmares are the only way for your shadow to get your attention. In Chapter Three, we'll explore how dreams that shock, disturb or haunt can be some of the most potent self-healing tools you'll ever receive.

Let's shine the night light now on the dark world of your shadow.

3

SHADOW DREAMING

We all dream of shadowy beasts and strangers and dark forces sometimes. And when we do, we tend to wake up shaken, disturbed or even ashamed. But those dreams – nightmares filled with looming unknown figures, horrifying events, monsters or troubling feelings – aren't always warnings from an external evil. Again, they are mirrors for personal and spiritual growth. They reflect a side of ourselves or a mindset we'd rather not look at, let alone claim. But this is exactly what these dreams are asking us to do. They are showing us that the aspects of ourselves that we repress are all too often projected onto others in our waking lives – and that projection can cause us great internal damage.

Welcome to the murky realm of your shadow self – the hidden, denied and often disowned parts of who we are. And nightmares, of course, are their playground.

Monsters

Imagine this: you're dreaming and in the dream you're stealing something. You feel a rush of adrenaline as you slip a ring into your pocket, looking over your shoulder, aware you're doing something wrong. Then someone confronts you. You lie. You spin stories to escape. You wake up in a cold sweat, disgusted with yourself and your unpleasant dream. 'Why would I dream something like that? That's not me.'

But what if it *is* you? Or at least, some hidden part of you? Perhaps you have previously adopted opinions or perspectives from others that aren't in line with your own values or are diminishing you in some way? This dream is not showing you the whole truth but pointing towards a piece of truth you've pushed into hiding or don't want to admit to.

We all have a shadow – however pious we may believe ourselves to be in our waking lives. It's made of the traits we reject in ourselves – jealousy, arrogance, selfishness, rage, neediness, envy and so on – and traits that society and our peers consider inappropriate. These are parts of ourselves that we've learned are unacceptable or unwise to express, so we may project those traits onto others and in the process banish them to our inner basement. But in dreams, that basement door swings wide open.

You see, dreams are many things but – as should be clear by now – they are above all shockingly honest. If the emperor has no clothes, they will point out that the emperor is naked when no one else has the courage to speak or see the truth behind what they are told by others. Even if they shock you, dreams will always speak your whole inner truth – of which your shadow side is a key part. And this key part will most clearly reveal itself in nightmares and sometimes in unwanted thoughts that break through during waking life.

Shadow dreams are not evidence that you're broken or 'bad'. They're simply signs that some part of your inner world urgently needs to be acknowledged, understood and reflected on with compassion, because the more you deny or repress it the more disconnected from your own soul you will become. The more empty, inauthentic and unfulfilled you will feel in waking life.

Shadow Work Is Deep

To truly know yourself – not just the parts you're proud of but also the hidden, messy, vulnerable aspects you wish weren't there – is the beginning of genuine personal and spiritual growth. This is not a journey of self-discovery in the traditional sense. It is a return. A sacred return to the fullness of who you are, to your soul, to your innate wholeness.

Why do we shy away from this inner work? Because the shadow – the parts of us we keep in the dark – feels frightening, shameful or unacceptable. But here's a truth that can help set you free: your shadow doesn't just hold your wounds or weaknesses; it also contains vast reservoirs of untapped creative energy, wisdom and resilience. Buried within what you've rejected are the very qualities that, when they are integrated, have the potential to transform your life.

Psychologist Carl Jung called this hidden treasure the 'golden shadow'. It is the brilliance you've pushed away because it didn't fit the version of you the world expected or the less-than version of you that you thought was essential for others to accept you. But what if those disowned parts are fragments of your inner gold? What if your envy points to unlived desires? Your anger to a suppressed voice? Your shame to a need for greater authenticity?

Take, for example, someone who deeply craves attention but judges this craving as selfish or vain. To be accepted, they bury the desire. But in doing so they also suppress the natural gifts that come with it – perhaps a gift for performance, leadership or storytelling. When this longing is denied, it festers into self-sabotage or low self-worth. But when brought into conscious awareness and embraced with compassion, it becomes a source of power, purpose and even joy.

Lizzy's Frenemy Shadow Dream

Now consider a woman, 'Lizzy', haunted by a disturbing recurring dream in which she kills her best friend. The emotional aftermath was intense: horror, guilt, confusion. What kind of person dreams such horrific things? But through gentle dreamwork and shadow exploration, a deeper truth emerged. Her friend in the dream symbolized all the polished traits the dreamer felt pressured to display themselves – perfection, success, social charm. The act of killing wasn't about her friend at all; it was about releasing the false self she had constructed to maintain that friendship.

Beneath Lizzy's guilt lay profound relief. Her dream was a message from her soul, urging her to stop performing and start being herself. When she allowed herself to acknowledge her real emotions – jealousy, insecurity, grief – something unexpected happened. She didn't lose her friend. She found herself.

This is the dark alchemy of shadow work. It transforms the monsters in your dreams into messengers, the fear into fuel, the darkness into depth. It is not always easy, but it is always sacred. Because every part of you, even the parts you hide, is trying to lead you out of the shadows towards your own inner light.

You Are Not Your Shadow

When a shocking dream paints you as a liar, a cheat, a coward, a thief or even something darker, like a murderer or criminal, it can shake you to your core. The emotional sting is sharp. Your first instinct may be to recoil and defend: 'That's not who I am!' But instead of rejecting the image outright, what if you paused and asked, 'What part of me does this represent? What if this uncomfortable vision isn't an accusation but an opportunity to understand myself better?'

Nightmares don't come to shame you. They come to wake you up in more ways than the literal. They aren't judgements passed down from some inner jury. Rather, they are urgent messages from your psyche and soul, challenging you to become more aware of conflict in your internal landscape. You are not defined by your shadow, nor by the darkness you see in your dreams – but you are deeply shaped by how you choose to react and relate to it. Will you face it with courage and curiosity? Or will you run from it, only to meet it again in your extreme dreams?

That's why, in the final chapter of this book, you'll find a list of 101 of the most-reported nightmare scenarios along with some simple tools to begin decoding them. In almost every case, the nightmare stems from the shadow self – the denied, ignored or misunderstood parts of your psyche. These dreams highlight our very human tendency to criticize or blame others for what we haven't yet made peace with inside ourselves.

It's important to remember that not all shadow dreams wear the mask of horror. Sometimes, your shadow expresses its pain in whimpers rather than screams. You might dream of being stuck in the passenger seat of a car, watching helplessly as someone else drives towards a cliff edge. You ask where you're going, but the driver doesn't respond. You feel frustrated, helpless, out of control. That dream is not just a surreal drama – it's a direct metaphor for your life. Perhaps you're surrendering your direction to others, drifting through your days without clear intention, allowing circumstances or other people's decisions to dictate your path.

Your inner world is speaking here through symbols. The message is simple but profound: take the wheel; reclaim your agency. Your life is not a ride you're meant to passively endure. It's a journey you are here to direct, not delegate to others. The road ahead may be uncertain, but the steering and the direction you set belongs to you.

Shadow work, then, is all about transformation. It's about learning to recognize the gold hidden in the darkness and realizing that you are always the one holding the key. When you accept that your shadow is part of you and that, just as day needs night, you can't exist or feel whole without it, you unlock the possibility of living with greater freedom, honesty and love.

Projection: The Shadow in Others

A curious and uncomfortable truth that often goes unspoken is that what we most dislike in others is often a reflection of what we find hard to accept in ourselves. When someone's words, actions or energy triggers a strong reaction in us, it may be more than a clash of personalities. It may be our shadow calling for attention. The psychological term for this is 'projection', a concept developed by Carl Jung to describe the way we unconsciously offload on to others the parts of ourselves that we don't want to own.

In Jung's words, 'The most dangerous psychological mistake is the projection of your own shadow onto others; this is the root of almost all conflicts.' In simpler terms, what you disown within yourself will often show up in your outer world, disguised as someone else's flaw. Those people who irritate, upset or trigger you may all be holding up a mirror to parts of yourself that remain unacknowledged.

Rather than face a difficult truth about who we are or what we feel, we assign that quality to someone else. In doing so, we avoid the inner discomfort of self-confrontation, at least temporarily. But projection isn't a permanent escape. It's a deflection that eventually returns to us without filters, often in chilling and disturbing dreams.

Kai's Mob Projection

Imagine a man, 'Kai', who dreams that he's being chased by an angry mob. They are yelling at him, calling him arrogant, self-righteous and dangerous. In the dream, he is terrified, convinced that if they catch him they will destroy him. The fear is visceral. The threat feels real. And yet, in his waking life, Kai prides himself on being humble, fair-minded and even-tempered. He's not the type to make a scene or seek the spotlight. But he's also highly critical of others, especially those who appear overly confident or assertive. He finds them abrasive – too much.

The dream brings him face to face with a difficult but liberating truth. The mob is not an external force. It is a manifestation of his own suppressed feelings, an internal uprising of the shadow voice he has silenced within himself. He's not being hunted by strangers. He's being hunted by the parts of himself he has rejected: the part that wants to be seen, to speak up, to express bold opinions. Instead of acknowledging that need, he has projected it onto others and judged them for owning what he cannot.

When Kai understands this, a door opens. He begins to experiment with expressing himself more honestly. He allows himself to speak up more in meetings, to offer ideas without apologizing, to stop defaulting to quiet agreement. He doesn't become arrogant; he becomes honest. And as he does so, his private judgement of others softens. Why? Because he no longer needs to project his discomfort onto them. He has claimed what was his all along.

This is the transformative power of recognizing projection for what it is: not a condemnation of your character but a need to look deeper at yourself. Your dreams dramatize this process in startling ways, but they always carry a hidden grace. They are inviting you to reclaim the energy you've given away – to stop fearing or condemning the traits you see in others and instead explore what those traits might be trying to tell you about yourself.

In this light, projection isn't a flaw. It's a compass. It points you towards the very places within that are ready for healing. And by acknowledging and integrating these parts, you not only grow in self-awareness but also begin to relate to others with more compassion, humility and clarity. Because in truth, the shadow you see in others might just be your own inner lighthouse, waiting to guide you to safety.

Dreams and Integrity

Sometimes, in dreams, we find ourselves doing things we would never imagine doing in waking life – lying, stealing, cheating or behaving in ways that challenge our moral compass. These dreams can be deeply unsettling, not because they predict our downfall but because they reveal subtle cracks between who we believe we are and how we're actually showing up, consciously or otherwise.

Remember: these dreams aren't judgement and punishment. They aren't proof that you're a bad person. Rather, they are invitations from your deeper self to realign. Your dream-self acts out scenarios that highlight a misalignment between your inner truth and your outer behaviour. In this sense dreams are like emotional and spiritual GPS alerts, quietly (and sometimes dramatically) whispering: 'You're drifting off course. Come back.'

Olivia's Relationship Reckoning

One woman, 'Olivia', shared a dream in which she was sneaking out behind her husband's back to meet a mysterious stranger for sex. The dream was charged with excitement but also thick with guilt. In waking life, she was engaging in what she called a harmless flirtation, convincing herself it wasn't serious. But the dream didn't let her hide. It stripped away her rationalizations and showed her the raw emotional betrayal already unfolding. The dream wasn't sentencing her – it was protecting her. It was asking Olivia to get honest with herself and make a conscious choice: either heal the cracks in her current relationship or leave it with integrity.

In their own dark and dramatic way, nightmares are wise guides. As I've mentioned previously, nightmares – and especially nightmares that come from the shadow – are course correctors, flashing messages from your soul that illuminate the growing distance between your deeper values and your actions. They challenge you to grow in integrity, to evolve towards the most honest and aligned version of yourself. When you listen to them with courage, they will always show you the way home.

Acting Out

Some dreams don't stay confined to the mind. They break through the veil of sleep and find expression in the physical world. Sleepwalking. Sleep talking. Crying out. Moving limbs. Even mimicking complex actions. This is where dreams become more than symbolic, they become embodied. And while these experiences can be disturbing to witness or endure, they are often signs of an underlying sleep disorder, especially when the brain fails to fully activate the natural paralysis that typically occurs during REM sleep.

Sleep talking can be startling. A person may mutter incoherently, shout vivid obscenities or even confess shocking things they would never say aloud while awake. These vocalizations might seem bizarre or deeply revealing but they are not conscious communications. They are often the brain's raw, unfiltered way of releasing emotional tension or processing unresolved feelings in the subconscious. In some cases, especially among older adults, these episodes can be an early sign of neurological conditions such as dementia. That's why any consistent or alarming disruption in sleep behaviour should always be taken seriously and discussed with a qualified medical professional.

From a scientific perspective, these nocturnal behaviours are typically viewed as stress responses or misfiring neural patterns. From a spiritual and psychological lens, they may be seen as a kind of dream catharsis – an involuntary release of inner chaos that the waking self has been unable or unwilling to express.

However, there are extreme and rare cases that go beyond catharsis, where dream enactment enters dangerous territory. In legal history, there have been genuine cases of individuals committing acts of violence, including assault and, tragically, even homicide, while asleep. These individuals were later found to have parasomnias or other serious sleep disorders and often had no memory of their actions. Such 'a dream made me do it' cases raise the question of whether someone can be held responsible for what they do while they are dreaming. Courts must rely on careful medical and psychological evaluations to navigate this legal and ethical grey area.

But one truth remains constant: dreams have immense power. Not only to move you emotionally and stir your soul but also to influence your body and behaviour. When the boundary between dreaming and waking begins to blur – when dreams spill into reality in ways that feel dangerous, disorienting or unmanageable – that's a clear signal to seek professional medical help.

This book honours the power of dreams as a sacred tool for transformation, insight and healing. But when dreams impact your safety or the safety of others, it's time to look beyond inner reflection and turn to medical and psychological expertise. There is no shame in this, only more wisdom. Recognizing when dreamwork is no longer solely a spiritual or psychological path but a health issue is itself an act of deep self-awareness.

Intrusive Thoughts: The Daytime Shadow

Although your shadow self is most likely to emerge in dreams or nightmares, be mindful that it can also surface during your waking hours as sudden, unwanted thoughts. These are the fleeting, often shocking ideas that seem to come out of nowhere. Picture this: you're standing on a train platform and a voice inside you murmurs, 'What if I jumped?' Or you're chopping vegetables and a flash of horror crosses your mind: 'What if I hurt someone I love?'

These are intrusive thoughts. They are deeply unsettling, but they are also deeply human. Again: you are not broken or dangerous for having them. You are not secretly evil. You're simply human with a complex, layered and ferociously curious experimental mind.

Sigmund Freud once interpreted these death drives as expressions of repressed instincts that clashed with societal norms. But modern psychology takes a more grounded view. Intrusive thoughts happen to everyone. What matters is not that you have them but how you respond to them. The danger is not in the thought itself but in attaching meaning to it that doesn't belong.

These thoughts are not intentions. They're not predictions or premonitions. They are fragments of your inner world rising to the surface, often because something inside you wants to shift, release or be acknowledged. Fear, desire, anger, chaos – these are all natural aspects of the psyche. The key is that you learn to witness these thoughts without fear or shame. Intrusive thoughts and death wishes are the mind's way of signalling emotional distress, not a true desire to die. They are mental alarms that something inside needs care or change.

Instead of recoiling or judging yourself harshly, pause and gently ask: 'What is this thought trying to show me? What unmet emotion or buried need lies beneath it?' These thoughts arise not because you wish harm but because something within you longs for change, for an ending, for transformation, for escape or simply for your attention.

The shadow is speaking. It is breaking through now from your dreams into your conscious life. Are you listening?

Often, your shadow will loosen its grip when you choose to stay present and enter a quiet, compassionate dialogue with it, without fear or judgement. When you meet these thoughts with understanding rather than resistance, they lose their power. The act of seeing them for what they are – as messengers, not monsters – is healing in itself.

True strength isn't about never having dark or difficult thoughts. It's about choosing love over fear, repeatedly, even in the face of your own inner shadows.

Your Inner Child

In essence, nightmares are not random but are urgent messages from the parts of ourselves we have pushed into the shadows during the day. But before launching into some shadow-work tools and techniques, it is important to reference another powerful Jungian psychological concept that can surface in nightmare scenarios – the inner child.

The inner child is the part of your psyche that still holds the emotional experiences, memories and needs of your early years. It is not just a symbol. It is a very real psychological and emotional presence within you. This inner child carries your joys, imagination and capacity for wonder as well as your unmet needs, fears and wounds from childhood. When those early emotional experiences are not fully acknowledged or healed, they don't simply vanish with age; they go underground into the unconscious mind. From there, the inner child continues to influence your behaviour, relationships and emotional reactions – often in ways you may not fully understand. Tuning into the inner child is not about regressing into immaturity but rather about reclaiming the vulnerable, feeling parts of yourself that were once silenced, shamed or abandoned. Healing begins when we turn towards that child within with wonder, compassion and a willingness to listen.

In Jungian terms, the inner child often lurks in the shadow – the unconscious realm that holds all that we have disowned. When the inner child is ignored for too long, it doesn't go silent. It grows restless, erupting in our nightmares, demanding to be acknowledged. Night terrors, recurring childhood settings or dreams of abandonment or helplessness can all be signs that the inner child is crying out from the shadow, asking you to turn towards the pain you once had no power to face and to acknowledge and nurture that inner child, parent it yourself now.

This is why inner-child work and shadow work are deeply entwined. Shadow work helps us to recognize the (typically negative) parts of ourselves that we've exiled and the inner child is often among the first to be cast out, deemed too needy, too sensitive, too much. By revisiting these aspects with compassion instead of judgement, we begin to transform what once haunted us.

Anna's Back-to-School Nightmare

Consider the story of 'Anna', a woman plagued by a recurring nightmare in which she wandered a school hallway, lost and crying while faceless adults ignored her. Through dreamwork and guided regression, Anna realized that the dream echoed a real-life memory of being left at school for hours as a child, feeling forgotten, because her mother could not pick her up on time. That experience had never been fully processed and her adult self had built walls around the vulnerability it caused. As Anna began to acknowledge the pain of her younger self, emotionally and intellectually, her nightmares stopped. The inner child didn't want to ruin her sleep; it just wanted to be seen and held.

So, nightmares don't just want us to confront the darkness; they want us to recover.

Losing Fear of the Dark

Ultimately, what most of us fear isn't the nightmare, or the intrusive thought, or even the shadow itself. What we truly fear is being left alone with ourselves – no noise, no screens, no distractions. Just us, sitting in stillness with our own unfiltered thoughts and feelings. That's where the real discomfort lies.

We fear the dark not because it is evil but because it is honest. It strips us bare and removes our masks. In the silence of night, in the depth of dreams, in the hush between heartbeats, we meet the unvarnished truth of who we really are – and often, that truth is not the polished version of ourselves that we present to the world. But this encounter is not something to dread. It is sacred. It is the very ground upon which all personal growth is built.

To fear your shadow is, at its heart, to fear your own power. To run from your nightmares is to silence the most instinctive part of your psyche – your soul trying to speak in a language beyond words. But when you turn towards the darkness with inquisitiveness instead of judgement, with compassion instead of resistance, you begin to reclaim parts of yourself you didn't even know were missing. These are your lost gifts, your own hidden strength, your own untapped wisdom.

The shadow-work practices at the end of this chapter are not meant to fix you. You're not broken, just a work in constant progress. They're here to help you soften your fear of your dreams, of your emotions, of the unknown places inside you. Because the truth is this: nightmares, intrusive thoughts and shadow dreams are not signs of spiritual failure. They are signs you are ready to learn and grow.

The question is no longer 'Why is this happening to me?' but 'What is this trying to awaken within me?'

Personal growth does not arise from always feeling good or staying in the light. That illusion is not healing; it's edging towards toxic positivity, a denial of your full human experience. Real growth begins when you stop pretending everything is okay and start leaning into the discomfort, allowing the dark to be your teacher.

Because the dark is not the opposite of light – it's the womb of it, where all creation begins. And when you choose to grow in the fertile soil of your own shadow, you don't just survive the night; you rise from it with renewed strength and power.

Shadow-Work Tools and Techniques: Dreaming Through Your Darkness

Remember: your shadow is not your enemy. It's a part of you that's been waiting patiently for acknowledgement, not to harm or control you but to reintegrate with the whole of who you are and to remind you that growth peaks in the darkness, where all untapped potential exists. These tools are designed to help you navigate that journey through extreme dreamwork and conscious reflection, so you can not only lose your fear of the dark but also learn to walk through it with anticipation.

Reclaim the dark: a night-facing ritual

This exercise will help you lose fear of the dark and begin building comfort with your own inner world. Fear of the dark often masks a deeper fear: fear of the unknown within us and fear of being alone. To do shadow work, you must be willing to sit in that discomfort and find peace there.

- Each evening when night falls, turn off all lights, switch your phone to silent and sit alone in complete darkness for five minutes.
- Keep your eyes open. Sit or lie comfortably. Breathe deeply.
- Allow thoughts, sensations or fears to surface. Do not try to change or fix anything. Just witness your thoughts and remind yourself that just because you think or feel something does not mean those thoughts and feelings define you.
- Whisper aloud: 'I am safe in the dark. I am safe in solitude. I welcome myself home.'
- After five minutes, write down what surfaced. Was it restlessness? A memory? Nothing at all? Don't judge those feelings. Simply notice them. Keep a log for seven nights.

- Over time, increase your getting comfortable alone in the dark time to ten or more minutes. You're training your nervous system to remain calm in the unknown. You're also proving to your own subconscious that you can be alone with your own thoughts and shadows and that nothing terrible happens when you do.

The shadow lens: identifying the shadow in your dreams

Every dream you have is a story woven from the threads of your subconscious and some of those threads are dark, tangled and uncomfortable to face. That's your shadow speaking. The shadow holds not only your fears and rejections but also your unlived potential, your raw instincts and the parts of you that never had the chance to be seen or accepted. Often, the shadow shows up as the villain, the monster, the stranger or the humiliated version of you in a dream. These characters are not external enemies; they are inner reflections, symbolizing the aspects of yourself that have been denied, hidden or pushed into the background.

This exercise helps you gently begin to identify and interpret the shadow symbols in your dreams so you can work with them, rather than against them.

- Choose a recent dream or nightmare that left you feeling disturbed, confused or emotionally charged. Look especially for dreams where someone is chasing you, attacking you, humiliating you or confronting you.

- List all the major characters in the dream. Include people, animals and even inanimate objects if they had a strong presence or personality.
- For each character, ask: 'What trait does this figure embody that bothers, frightens or embarrasses me? Do they remind me of someone in my life or a part of myself I try to suppress?'
- Now, turn the lens inward: 'Where in my life might I carry this same trait even subtly, even unconsciously? When have I felt the urge to behave this way but didn't let myself?'
- Gently reflect on your answers. This is not about self-blame; it's about self-integration. You're not looking for flaws; you're looking for truth and truth leads to wholeness.
- Optional: journal a dialogue between your waking self and one of the shadow characters. Ask them why they appeared. Let them speak freely, without censorship. You may be surprised by what they reveal.

The parts of yourself that you reject don't disappear – they return, repeatedly, in dreams and projections. By consistently meeting your shadow with curiosity and compassion in your dreamwork, you take the first step towards becoming whole. Remember: the shadow isn't here to terrify or hurt you. It's here to help you see what you've been brave enough to feel and dream about but haven't felt ready to face with your eyes wide open – until now.

Reclaiming your inner child through dream symbols

Your inner child, the part of you that still feels deeply, loves freely, fears abandonment and longs for unconditional safety often appears in your dreams in symbolic or distorted forms. Nightmares can be rich with inner-child wounding: abandonment, shame, fear of punishment or feeling unseen or unheard. But rather than pushing these dreams away, you can use them to reconnect with and begin healing the tender, innocent part of you that still lives within.

This exercise is about shifting your perspective and seeing your dreams, no matter how frightening, through the eyes of your inner child and offering them and yourself the love and understanding they and you once needed but perhaps never received.

- Choose a recent dream or nightmare where you, a character, an object or a place felt small, afraid, neglected, rejected or overwhelmed. Look for dreams where you were lost, ignored, trapped, punished or desperately trying to get someone's attention or approval. Look for dreams that feature babies and children, whether human or animal.

- Identify the emotional tone of the dream. What emotions were you feeling? Were you scared, sad, ashamed, helpless? These feelings may be echoes of your younger self, still living inside you.
- Now ask: 'In this dream, where might my inner child be present?'

  Are you the child in the dream? Is there a child in the dream you're trying to protect or ignore? Is there an adult who scares, neglects or abandons you?
- Next, visualize or write a letter from your adult self to the inner child in the dream.

  Tell them they are safe now. Acknowledge what they felt. Offer them the love, protection or validation they didn't get in the dream or perhaps in real life.
- Reimagine the dream with a different ending. Let your adult self enter the dream and comfort the child, confront the villain or change the outcome. This helps rewire your relationship with fear and powerlessness.
- Reflect: what does this child still need from you in waking life? More play? More rest? Less judgement? More permission to feel?

Your nightmares can be messages from a younger version of you, calling out across time for connection, comfort and healing. When you turn towards those cries with compassion, you don't just reclaim your inner child; you begin to parent yourself in the way you always needed. Healing doesn't mean erasing the past. It means loving yourself through revisiting it with understanding and compassion for the person you once were.

Befriend discomfort: get comfortable being uncomfortable

To help you embrace emotional discomfort in dreams, rather than escaping or repressing it, try this exercise. It will underline that growth happens only when you stop avoiding the hard parts. Discomfort is not your enemy – it's your guide.

- Before sleep, say to yourself: 'Tonight, I welcome any part of myself that wants to speak through my dreams, even if it makes me uncomfortable.'
- When you wake up from a difficult or uncomfortable dream, don't distract yourself. Sit with it.
- Write down three emotions the dream brought up. Then write: 'What do these feelings remind me of in waking life?' Note down any answers that come to mind.
- Breathe deeply and say aloud: 'These feelings are allowed. These parts of me are welcome as they have something of value to teach me. I will observe but not identify with them.'
- Moving forward: when you feel uncomfortable or fearful in your waking or dreaming life, transform that into excitement. It is a sign you are shedding old skins

(sometimes growth hurts) and ready to become a higher version of yourself.

Each time you do this exercise, you're building resilience from the inside out. Discomfort becomes a signpost for transformation ahead, not a red flag.

Spotting projection

To help you identify when you're projecting your shadow onto others – whether in dreams or in waking life – this technique will show you just how much psychological projection distorts your perception and damages relationships. Owning your projections sets you free.

- Think of a recent dream where someone annoyed, hurt or threatened you. Or think of a person in waking life you strongly dislike.
- Write down the exact qualities that upset you. Be specific: 'loud', 'manipulative', 'self-centred' and so on.
- Now ask yourself, being as honest as you can: 'When have I shown this trait? When have I feared others seeing this trait in me?'
- Sit with the discomfort. Breathe. If needed, journal a few sentences about how this trait might have once protected you or served a purpose in your past.
- How does potentially possessing this trait make you feel? Locate the emotion in your body.

- Once located, send feelings of unconditional love to this trait because it likely began with noble intention to keep you feeling safe. Let it know that it has done a great job, but you don't need it anymore and are ready to let it go.
- Now send feelings of unconditional love to a person in your waking life who triggers you. You may find this hard, if feelings run deep, and it may take some practice, but it is worth the effort because often when you change your perception of someone their power over you diminishes. And yes, people you have a grudge against do have an energetic unseen hold over you because you are giving them your attention. And where your attention goes, your energy flows.

Consciously choosing to send love to yourself and to someone who triggers you is mighty empowering and liberating. You take your own power back. Remember you don't project what you hate – you projected what you've disowned.

Rewrite the nightmare

This method has been used successfully to ease recurring nightmares by consciously rewriting them. It is based on therapeutic techniques used for PTSD and trauma. Indeed, PTSD studies have shown that rescripting nightmares when awake can reduce emotional distress and even stop the dreams entirely. This technique is used in imagery rehearsal therapy (IRT).

- Choose a nightmare that repeats or carries intense fear.
- Write it down in full, detail by detail, however unpleasant.
- Now, rewrite it as if you are in control – because, news flash, you are! Keep the structure and opening scenario of the nightmare but change your reactions and the outcome so it is in your favour. For example, if you were chased, now you turn and speak to the chaser. If you were helpless, now you find your strength. If there were beasts, transform them into butterflies.
- Before sleep, read your new version. Visualize it or feel it playing out with you in control of how it manifests this time.

Repeat this exercise until the nightmare loses its hold over you – and it will, because your brain begins to emotionally reprocess the fear through scripting the nightmare. The dream may transform or fade. More importantly, you reclaim authorship over your inner world. You remind yourself that nightmares don't happen to you. They are created by you, for you and are all about you.

Daylight shadows: working with unwanted thoughts

Try this exercise to bring compassion and understanding to intrusive thoughts that may arise during the day. It will help reinforce the idea that intrusive thoughts are normal. What matters is how you respond to them – not their content.

- The next time you have a disturbing thought – 'What if I jumped?' or 'What if I hurt someone?' – pause.
- Say silently: 'That was just a thought passing through and not a truth or my identity. My shadow is speaking. What does it want me to understand better?'
- Ask yourself what feeling might this thought be trying to express. Fear? Stress? Desire for escape? Anger?
- Finally, write this question in your journal: 'If this thought had a helpful message for me, what might it be?' Again, if any answers come to mind, note those down too.

Never forget that you are not your thoughts and you are not your feelings. You are your choices. The thought is not you. It's just a signal. When you choose to meet it with fascination instead of fear, it softens and, in that softening, brings you closer to illumination.

Whole Again

The shadow is in the business not of shaming you but of shaping you. Bad dreams, nightmares and strange thoughts when you are awake don't mean something's wrong with you. They mean something is trying to surface, be understood and become whole. By meeting your shadow – through dreamwork, honest reflection and a healthy dose of self-compassion and curiosity – you reclaim your own lost energy, creativity and truth.

You become someone who is no longer afraid of the dark, because you've made peace with what lives there. You become someone who is comfortable being alone, because you know the template for all your other relationships is the one you have with yourself. If that self-relationship is respectful and compassionate, this is the kind of relationship you are likely to attract.

After reading this chapter, the next time you wake from a frightening dream, I gently invite you not to turn away too quickly. Don't rush to suppress or forget what you've seen or felt. Instead, take a sacred pause. Breathe. Soften. Listen. What if this fearsome dream isn't a tormentor but a teacher in disguise? What if something deep within you is reaching out not to punish or frighten you but to offer you a forgotten truth?

As dreadful as they seem, nightmares often emerge at a time in your life when your soul is ready or longing to grow. They pull aside the veil of your everyday persona and reveal what you've hidden – not because you are weak but because you are finally strong enough to take a look. You are so much more than the polished identity you show to the world. You are layered, luminous and limitless. You are the calm and the chaos, the light and the shadow.

Darkness has its own beauty, if only we dare to see it. Just as it is only in the velvet hush of night that the brightest stars appear, so too it is often in your darkest dreams that your deepest healing begins. The night doesn't come to consume your light; it comes to remind you that you always carry its potential within. And those stars? They don't just shine despite the darkness they shine because of it. So, the next time your shadow finds you, in your dream or in your waking life, meet it with fascination and wonder. It might just be the beginning of becoming whole and truly knowing yourself for the first and not the last time.

4

LIMINAL DREAMING

Caution: this chapter is intentionally crafted to reflect the liminal shifting themes it explores. For your safety, please do not engage with it while driving or operating machinery.

To fully experience its effect, slow down and read it (out loud if you can) or listen to it mindfully. Let each sentence settle. When you reach the end, resist the urge to rush headfirst into the next chapter. Instead, pause. Take a few long, slow breaths. Close your eyes. Notice what images begin to stir behind them and what rises from the stillness.

And if you find yourself drifting towards sleep at any point when you read or listen to this chapter and a ten- or twenty-minute nap feels like what you need, then give yourself permission to take it. Find a quiet, safe space to lie down and let go. Napping isn't just rest. It's one of the most direct and powerful ways to enter, explore and engage with the transformative potential of the liminal dream space.

There is a moment just before you fall asleep and another one immediately on waking – slippery, twilight and easily forgotten – when consciousness begins to dissolve and extreme visions can sometimes surface behind your eyes. It's not quite sleep, not quite wakefulness. It's a borderland between worlds, a dreamlike space where thought turns fluid and the mind unbuttons from its usual tight attire. These two states are not just fleeting curiosities. They are volatile, highly impressionable and sometimes petrifying arenas of dreamlike perception. In sleep science and dream research, they are called the 'liminal states'.

The first liminal state, called hypnagogia, is the transitional state from wakefulness into sleep. The second liminal state, hypnopompia, occurs from sleep back into waking. Though brief, these passages are intensely fertile states of consciousness, rich with sensory distortion, vivid imagery, fractured narratives and the potential for profound emotional or spiritual awareness. Strange sights, disembodied voices, jolting sensations or uncanny presences are not uncommon. These shapeshifting moments can hold raw emotional charge – fear, awe, wonder – and, significantly, can often contain the same kinds of frightening imagery that populates our nightmares.

It's important to understand from the outset that these liminal states offer the two most powerful windows or bridges to connect with your dreaming mind and waking intuition and therefore to understand and transform the nightmares that may arise or be summoned up by them. Just as nightmares are messages encoded in intense emotional symbolism, these liminal-state statements can crack open the seal between conscious and unconscious experience. They too can bring buried content that needs to be understood and noticed to the surface. They are, in many ways, the gateways through which nightmares can slip in or out.

But as with any threshold, they can feel uncanny. The liminals are not entirely under our control. We do not step into them like a familiar room. We fall, drift or are pulled into or out of them. Sometimes we are aware of them, but most of the time we are not. This unpredictability can be unsettling. Many people report sensations of being watched, of presence in the room or of falling through space. Others may experience paralysis during these transitions, where the mind is aware but the body is not yet responsive – an especially common context for frightening visions and waking nightmares.

To explore these states and their serious personal-growth potential, we must first understand what happens when the mind shuts down its usual processing in preparation for sleep and the body enters a kind of rehearsed, nightly paralysis. The brain does not simply go offline during sleep. Instead, it enters cycles of activity that open access to parts of ourselves we rarely meet in waking life. In these fragile, flickering borderlands, the veil between inner and outer worlds thins, just as it is believed on Halloween the veil between this life and the afterlife thins.

Drifting into Hypnagogia: The Descent Begins

Falling asleep is not a switch being flipped. It's a gradual process, a series of sliding panels that quietly close one after the other. As the body begins to relax and the metabolic rate drops, the brain shifts its rhythm, winding down the higher-frequency beta waves of alertness into slower alpha waves associated with relaxation. Soon, these are replaced by the even slower theta waves of Stage 1 sleep. This is the entryway into the dreamworld: it's not a door we walk through but one we drift across almost unknowingly.

And there is a tantalizing moment, just before sleep truly takes hold, when we are still aware just enough. In this state, our thoughts become less linear. Images begin to arise, strange and often fleeting. These images aren't always coherent and they don't follow the narrative logic of full dreaming. They can be abstract – a floating shape, a burst of colour, a voice murmuring nonsense or a memory that morphs into something unrecognizable. Sometimes they are jarring: a face melting, a sudden jolt, a sensation of falling.

This is not yet full-blown dreaming, but the architecture of dreams begins here. What we experience during hypnagogia may seem random but it is never meaningless. It's as if the unconscious mind is warming up its language – symbols, images, emotions and questions – before fully transitioning into the dream state.

Because hypnagogia occurs in the theta brainwave state, it is also highly impressionable. This is the same state young children spend much of their time in, which is why negative words spoken to a child can be so damaging: they imprint directly onto the developing brain, making them difficult to reprogramme later in life.

In a similar way, what you tell yourself just before falling asleep is deeply influential. Your thoughts at this threshold moment go straight into your subconscious. That's why setting dream intentions, or practising gratitude before sleep and immediately upon waking, can be so transformative. The liminal states offer two of the most powerful opportunities each day to shift negative thought patterns and beliefs into more positive ones. It also explains the truth behind the old saying that you should never go to sleep on an argument.

Many of us have experienced the hypnic jerk, that sudden twitch or sensation of tripping over the edge of something. This is hypnagogia's calling card. The body, unsure if it's sleeping, sometimes misfires and flinches. Evolutionarily, some scientists believe it may be a primitive survival mechanism, the brain's way of checking if the body is still safe before surrendering to physical paralysis.

Artists, writers and mystics have long courted this liminal state for its surreal creativity and the preview it offers to the contents of your dreaming mind. But, as previously mentioned, it is also an unpredictable space where savage visions can arise – startling faces, disembodied voices, sounds with no source. Because hypnagogia lacks the escapism of dreams or the rational control of wakefulness, it often feels unsettling. One does not watch these visions. One is conscious inside them.

It is precisely this immersive quality that gives hypnagogia its power and, at times, its terror. In the context of nightmares, these early-sleep visions can be the seeds of nocturnal fear, shaping the emotional tone of what follows on in our dreams. The boundary is thin. Most of the time we fall asleep swiftly and aren't even aware of the hypnogogic state, but sometimes, the nightmare begins before we've even fallen asleep.

Hypnopompia: The Rise Back Through Shadow

On the other side of sleep is hypnopompia, the state of awakening. Often softer and more gradual and less creatively rich than hypnagogia, it is nonetheless awash with strange phenomena. As we come out of REM sleep, where most vivid dreaming occurs, the brain can sometimes wake up before the body does. This occasional misalignment between mental awareness and physical immobility allows fragments of the dreamworld to linger on as we open our eyes.

In hypnopompia, we may still hear voices, feel presences or perceive visual hallucinations, even though we are technically awake. The dream residue bleeds into the room. Sounds may echo with no source. Shadows may seem to breathe. Often, we are confused, uncertain of what is real and what is not. This uncanny blending of dream and waking perception can feel mystical, surreal or deeply unsettling.

This is particularly disorienting when accompanied by sleep paralysis of the body, an entirely natural, if terrifying, part of this liminal landscape. The body remains locked in the paralysis of REM sleep while the mind begins to stir. We may find ourselves unable to move or speak, caught in an eerie in-between, conscious but powerless. In this vulnerable state, the remnants of dreams can feel like menacing figures at the edge of the bed, whispers from unseen mouths, a weight on the chest.

For some, this is a fleeting curiosity. For others, especially those prone to nightmares, hypnopompia can become a repeating site of fear. What makes this state so powerful and so disturbing is its ambiguity and not knowing if you are asleep or awake. The rational mind has not yet fully returned, but the emotional and imaginative faculties remain wide open. It is here that unresolved psychic content can surface with urgency. The boundary between the inner world and the outer one has not yet reformed.

Just like hypnagogia, hypnopompia is not a mistake of the brain. It is a doorway – a transitional state that offers access and deeper insight to the hidden spaces of the psyche. And like any threshold, what emerges there can be illuminating or frightening. The visions are real in the way all emotions and inner experiences are real. They speak a language that can't be reasoned with, only witnessed. This fragile time between dreaming and waking holds deep significance. Sometimes, the nightmare does not end with sleep and anxious feelings and symbols from it follow us into waking. But just as easily, this state can be a place of insight, release and creative breakthrough, if we choose to engage with it rather than recoil.

REM Atonia

There remains a lot of confusion about the term 'sleep paralysis'. It sounds frightening – and for many of the people who have experienced it consciously, it is. But it's also one of the most misunderstood phenomena in sleep science. It is an entirely natural part of the falling asleep process and happens every single night, though most of aren't even aware of it. Sleep paralysis is a protective neurological mechanism that occurs during REM sleep – though I prefer its more poetic and evocative name, REM atonia, as it sounds far less alarming.

As mentioned above, your body becomes paralysed when you fall asleep to prevent you from physically acting out your dreams. The muscles go slack, voluntary control is suppressed and you become still as stone. This is not dangerous; in fact, it is essential for safe dreaming. Without REM atonia, we might flail, kick or sleepwalk during intensely vivid dreams, potentially harming ourselves or others. Indeed, when there are glitches in the REM atonia state – often triggered by waking stress and anxiety or a sleep disorder – this is when sleepwalking and talking may occur.

But, as already indicated, sometimes – especially during hypnopompia, the twilight state between sleep and wakefulness – our consciousness returns before the body unfreezes. We wake up mentally, but the body remains inert, locked in the temporary paralysis of REM. In this paralysis, people often report the inability to move or speak, a sense of weight on the chest, difficulty breathing and, most commonly, the sensation that something or someone is in the room. Often, this presence feels malevolent. Its arrival is accompanied by an overwhelming sense of dread. People describe it as being watched, hunted or even possessed.

Sleep paralysis has occurred throughout human history and across every known culture. And in nearly every account, it has a face – a folklore creature, a demonic force, an unwanted visitor from beyond the veil. In medieval Europe, it was said to be the work of an *incubus*, a male demon who sits on sleeping women, or a *succubus*, a female demon who seduces sleeping men. In Newfoundland, it's known as the 'Old Hag' sitting on your chest. In Japan, it is *kanashibari* being bound by an invisible force. In Nigeria, it might be seen as a spiritual attack from jealous enemies. In Brazil, the blame falls on

Pisadeira, an old woman who lurks on rooftops and walks on the chests of sleepers.

What all these stories have in common is a sense of heavy presence: someone else is there, intruding, pressing down, invading the sanctum of the sleeper. The universality of these reports suggests that the phenomenon has deep, perhaps primal, roots in human neurobiology, but the way it appears, the mask it wears, depends on the stories and metaphors our culture provides. It could explain many reports of hauntings and even cases of alien abduction.

Some cognitive studies suggest that these experiences may well be hallucinations generated by a half-dreaming brain struggling to make sense of sensory deprivation.* The mind, in a panic, projects meaning into silence and stillness. But knowing this – knowing the explanation – doesn't necessarily make the experience feel any less real. The terror feels real. The presence feels real. The memory lingers.

Sleep paralysis may be a neurological reality, but it also touches upon something ancient and is a place where fear and folklore meet in the threshold between worlds.

---

* Clemens Speth and Jana Speth, 'A New Measure of Hallucinatory States and a Discussion of REM Sleep Dreaming as a Virtual Laboratory for the Rehearsal of Embodied Cognition', *Cognitive Science*, 42(1) (2018), pp. 311–333, doi: 10.1111/cogs.12491.

Paul's Demonic Warning

Consider the strange dream case of Paul. He came to a sleep clinic after experiencing recurring demonic episodes that left him afraid to sleep alone. Paul described the events in detail: he would wake up in the middle of the night, unable to move, with a crushing weight on his chest. A shadowy figure – a woman with hollow eyes and a twisted smile – would straddle him, breathing hot breath into his face.

'She would lean in,' Paul said, 'and whisper things I didn't understand, in a language I've never heard. I couldn't scream. I couldn't breathe. Sometimes, it felt like she was pulling my soul out.'

Paul was raised Catholic and although he had drifted from religion, he believed these were real succubus or demonic attacks. He began researching exorcisms and visited a local priest who told him to sleep with a crucifix under his pillow.

The episodes continued. Eventually, Paul found his way to a sleep specialist who explained the phenomenon as sleep paralysis, specifically within the hypnopompic state. The dark woman was not a demon but a hallucinatory image created by his semi-lucid mind, still partly caught in REM, still paralysed by REM atonia. The feeling of being suffocated? A combination of shallow REM breathing and panicked awareness of immobility. The foreign whispers? Auditory remnants of a dream, interpreted by a brain desperate for explanation.

This knowledge helped Paul begin to contextualize his experiences. He started practising better sleep hygiene: consistent bedtime, reduced caffeine and alcohol and the elimination of screens an hour before sleep. More importantly, he began to reframe the episodes not as spiritual assaults but as misfiring sleep mechanisms. He also started to brainstorm the meaning of exorcism and look at areas of his life that he needed to let go of or release for his own wellbeing.

Over time, the frequency of the events lessened. When they did occur, Paul no longer panicked. 'I still see her sometimes,' he told the clinic six months later, 'but now I tell myself: this is entirely natural. And she fades. I also see it as a warning sign that I am not taking care of myself and I am letting negative thoughts take over again.'

Mirror, Mirror

Liminal dreaming, whether falling into sleep or rising from it, is yet another psychological mirror. It reflects not just the contents of our unconscious but our beliefs, fears and the cultural language we use to describe what is unknown beneath the surface. The images that appear in hypnagogia and hypnopompia are not random; they are shaped by our memory, expectation, trauma, desire. In these borderlands, our sense of self becomes porous. The guardrails of rationality are temporarily gone and through the cracks can slip angels or abominations.

But here's the key: these states are not pathological. Everyone experiences them to some degree. The bizarre, disjointed visions of hypnagogia, the lingering memories from dreams of hypnopompia and the scary paralysis of waking up mentally before the body does are all are a natural part of the normal architecture of human sleep. The danger lies not in the experience but in our interpretation of it and response to it.

When misunderstood, these states can feel like spiritual assaults, alien abductions or signs of madness. But when understood as a perfectly natural part of the sleeping and waking process, they offer insight into the dream-making creativity of the brain. They reveal how the unconscious speaks not in words but in symbols, sensations and archetypes. The shadowy woman at the foot of the bed is not a literal demon. She is a personification of fear, vulnerability and loss of control. The floating sensation is not your soul leaving your body; it is the detachment of your sensory network, momentarily disconnected from muscular feedback.

The liminal states do suggest that the boundaries of self are flexible and that reality is, at best, a negotiation between what we expect to perceive and what our mind constructs. In my opinion, these states are a nightly warmup act for the transformative and healing potential of the dream state and for entering a different stage of consciousness. They are as old as sleep itself and in their shadows we can see not just our fears but also our creativity, our memory and our longing for meaning rise to the surface and break through into our conscious awareness.

And perhaps most poignantly, these dream thresholds whisper that we are never truly alone. Within the seeming chaos of fragmented imagery and dreamlike logic lies an ancient intelligence, our inner oracle, offering metaphors instead of facts, sensations instead of sentences. If we approach these states with reverence rather than resistance, they can become sacred portals to healing, imagination and spiritual insight in much the same way as full-blown dreams can. The liminal is not a void but a vessel. It carries messages from the deep, coded in emotion and myth, inviting us to listen with our whole being and not just our waking mind.

Why It Feels So Real

One of the most jarring features of hypnagogic and hypnopompic states is the vividness of their imagery. They can feel so real. Unlike regular dreams, which often occur within deeper sleep and may dissolve like mist upon waking, liminal dreams do tend to imprint themselves with extraordinary clarity. This is because they happen so soon before we fully wake up, when the mind is more alert, more attuned and more susceptible to emotional flooding – a sudden rush of fear, awe, longing or even arousal. These experiences can arrive like waves, overwhelming the senses and bypassing logical filters, leaving behind a residue that can haunt or inspire us for days.

This is one reason why images experienced during sleep paralysis are so shocking. You are awake – or you believe you are – but unable to move. Your environment feels real: your room, the light, the sounds, the familiar textures of waking life. And yet something is subtly, deeply strange. The shadows breathe. A figure stands just outside your line of sight. You sense a presence. Breathing feels tight, as though the air itself is thick with meaning. Every fibre of your being screams that something unnatural is happening. And still, this is the body doing exactly what it was designed to do, remaining safely paralysed in REM atonia while the brain transitions between realms of consciousness.

The emotional intensity of these moments often convinces people they've had a supernatural encounter. And who is to say they haven't? The realm of the liminal does not distinguish easily between inner and outer, spirit and psyche. Many who experience hypnagogic visions resist scientific explanations not because they are irrational but because no clinical language captures the raw, mythic power of what they felt. This is the paradox: the closer we are to waking, the more convincing the dream becomes. These are not mere hallucinations – they are revelations, encoded in symbol and sensation.

Despite the fear they can evoke, hypnagogic and hypnopompic states are not enemies. They can become doors to creativity, healing and profound insight. Modern dreamwork, mindfulness practices and depth psychology are beginning to reclaim these states as gateways to deeper self-awareness.

If entered with reverence and wonder, hypnagogia becomes a sanctuary of imagination. It is a sacred in-between where the rational mind loosens its grip and the intuitive mind begins to speak. Thought and image dance together. In hypnopompia, too, the soul lingers, half-rooted in the dreamworld, half-reaching towards the light of day. Lucid dreamers (see page 167), visionaries and truth seekers of all kinds are learning to ride this delicate wave, drawing wisdom from the dark waters of the unconscious into the brightness of waking life.

Some of our most celebrated writers, artists and thinkers have dipped their brushes and pens into these liminal spaces. William Blake, Edgar Allan Poe and Mary Shelley were just a few of the creators drawn to the numinous and all were intimately familiar with this twilight edge of awareness and understood that the liminal states are not neurological anomalies. They are, in a very real sense, our most ancient muse, offering glimpses of the cosmos within and inviting us to listen to what the night mind longs to reveal.

Transforming the Threshold

Returning to Paul's story, outlined earlier in this chapter, there's something profoundly healing and revealing in how he began to reclaim his experience. The *succubus* did not vanish overnight. She still appeared in moments of stress or after too much caffeine. But it wasn't her presence that changed but rather Paul's relationship to the experience. What had once been a spine-chilling visitation began to soften at the edges, transforming from a threat to resist to a reminder to pause and reflect on where his current mindset was taking him.

This is the essence of nightmare transformation: not erasing the image, not forcing it away but confronting it with courage, curiosity, creativity and compassion. True healing begins when we stop running from the monster and instead ask it why it came to us. Nightmare therapy, lucid dreaming and liminal-dream practices invite the dreamer to turn inward and ask the shadow: 'Who are you?' And sometimes, astonishingly, it answers not in language but in subtle inner shifts of awareness. The demon becomes a frightened child. The weight on the chest transforms into unwept grief. The dark intruder at the door is revealed as a long-buried trauma, now rising into the light, seeking integration.

Like many others who walk the path of conscious dreamwork, Paul learned to name the experience: sleep paralysis, or REM atonia, or hypnopompic hallucination. Naming it gave him power. But even more than that, it gave him a sense of belonging. He was no longer a solitary sufferer in the night but part of a much larger story – a shared archetypal journey that spans centuries and cultures. He understood that people across the globe have encountered this same dark visitor, clothed in different forms but carrying the same symbolic weight.

When we view these encounters through the lens of liminal dreaming and what we understand about it, we realize that they are not random intrusions or signs of madness. They call us to confront the unacknowledged parts of ourselves, to step into the underworld of our psyche and to emerge changed. These shapeshifting images don't come to torment but instead to offer us passages.

To face what surfaces in the liminal states is to cross a threshold into deeper self-awareness. It is to reclaim the lost, the feared and the forgotten aspects of who we are. In this way, the hypnagogic state becomes instead a dark angel pointing the way to personal growth. Paul's story reminds us that transformation doesn't always mean eliminating the fear; it can mean finding the wisdom within it. Sometimes the most frightening images and sensations are the ones most urgently trying to help us wake up – not from sleep but into the fullness of our own being.

Guardians of the Threshold

The borderlands of hypnagogia and hypnopompia are strange, haunting and holy places. They are not just mechanical crossings. They are psychological thresholds: between control and surrender, between day and night, between self and shadow. They are liminal chambers of inner alchemy, where the soul loosens its grip on linear thought and slips into something older, wilder and infinitely wiser.

It is no surprise that our minds paint these liminal passages with such vivid colour. Here is where our hidden selves gather, like fog along the coast. Here is where ancient fears awaken. And here is where insight is born not through reason but through revelation. We don't solve mysteries here; we become them.

In a culture that values wakefulness, logic and productivity, these half-waking, half-dreaming states are often ignored, feared or dismissed. But perhaps we should learn to sit more willingly at the edge of sleep, not just as a retreat into rest but as an entry point into the mythic, the unconscious, the mysterious, the dreamworld. These spaces whisper secrets the daylight self cannot hear.

For in these moments, when the world fades and we are suspended between sleep and wake, we meet the guardians of the threshold – not demons, not angels but parts of ourselves that have been long unseen. They are the disguised faces of our own intuition, longing, grief and genius. They guard nothing but the truth we've been too busy or too frightened to hear.

And when we listen, truly listen, we may find they were never here to alarm us. They were simply waiting to be understood, to be welcomed and to prepare us for the infinite creativity we meet in our own dreams. Their presence marks the entrance to the sacred inner wilderness.

In essence, the liminal states are not haunted passageways. They are treasure chests of insight and creative potential. Here, in these thin spaces between waking and sleeping, lies a well of creativity waiting to be tapped. Neither chaotic nor random but rich with personal symbolism and archetypal resonance, these states connect us with a part of the psyche that never stops dreaming, even in waking life.

Few artists knew this better than Salvador Dalí, who developed a peculiar trick to catch inspiration in the very moment it appeared. He would sit in an armchair holding a large metal key or spoon in one hand, positioned just above a ceramic plate. As he began to drift into sleep, the muscles in his hand would relax, the key would fall, hit the plate with a loud clang and wake him. In those fractions of a second between alertness and dreaming, he would capture surreal, dream-charged images that became the seeds of many of his paintings.

The inventor Thomas Edison likewise kept ball bearings in his hand and let them drop into a metal tray as he nodded off. This wasn't just eccentric behaviour – it was a method of controlled hypnagogia. Both Dalí and Edison were harvesting the surreal just before slipping fully into unconsciousness.

This state – the moment when the body lets go and the mind begins to wander – offers a direct line to the unconscious mind. Images, sounds and feelings that we often can't access during waking life suddenly rise to the surface. And unlike full dreams, which are often forgotten, these fragments can be remembered with astonishing clarity, especially if we train ourselves to become aware of the liminal.

To honour these threshold moments is to honour the mystery at the heart of being human. For here, suspended between two worlds, the veil thins and through it creativity, wisdom and even healing may flow. And if after reading or listening to this you are eager to work with the liminal states, here are some reminders and practical tips to point you in the right direction.

Practical Steps for Navigating Liminal Dreaming

First and foremost, if you experience vivid hypnagogia, frightening hypnopompia or episodes of sleep paralysis, know this: you are not broken. You are not cursed. You are experiencing a natural, though often misunderstood, part of the human sleep cycle, one that has been misinterpreted for centuries because of its emotional intensity, symbolic resonance and surreal, sometimes terrifying, imagery.

These liminal states are not signs of dysfunction; they are spectacular invitations to deeper awareness. Your night mind is eager to draw your attention to what your waking self may have pushed aside. While the experiences can be overwhelming, they are also navigable and, in time, even transformative. Here are some approaches that can help:

1. **Sleep regularly and well.** Irregular sleep schedules and sleep deprivation increase the likelihood of sleep paralysis and unsettling liminal experiences. Establish a calming bedtime routine that signals to your body and mind that it's safe to let go. Avoid stimulants late in the day and aim for seven to nine hours of uninterrupted, nurturing sleep. Think of your sleep as a sacred practice – a return to the inner temple of the self.

2. **Track the experiences.** Document when liminal episodes occur, what you felt, what you saw and any physical or emotional conditions that preceded them. Are they more likely after emotional stress? Alcohol? Certain positions? Tracking patterns helps reclaim agency and reveals your personal symbolism.
3. **Change sleeping position.** Both research and anecdotal evidence suggest that sleep paralysis occurs more frequently when lying on your back. Simply shifting to a side-sleeping position can drastically reduce the frequency of episodes. Consider placing a pillow behind your back to keep yourself supported in a sideways posture throughout the night.
4. **Mindful acceptance.** If paralysis strikes, your instinct may be to panic but awareness is your ally. Focus on your breath. Try to wiggle a toe or finger – these small actions often interrupt the paralysis. Repeat a calming mantra, such as: 'This is my old friend REM atonia paying me a visit again. I am safe. This will pass.' The more calmly and consciously you respond, the less fearful the experience becomes over time.
5. **Reframe the imagery.** Instead of resisting or fearing the entities or sensations you perceive, consider approaching them with inquisitiveness as personal-growth tools. Ask inwardly: 'What are you here to teach me?' This question, posed with sincerity, can reframe the entire experience from one of terror to

> one of insight, even healing. Sometimes the demon is a disguised protector. Sometimes the fear is a veil over wisdom waiting to be revealed.

Above all, trust that these experiences, though intense, are part of your mind's vast, creative terrain. With time, practice and compassionate self-enquiry, the liminal realm can become less of a battlefield and more of a library. You are not lost in the dark. You are learning to see deep into yourself in a new kind of light.

Becoming Conscious in Your Sleep

One of the most thrilling and profound potentials of becoming aware during these borderland states is the gateway they offer into lucid dreaming, those extraordinary experiences in which you not only know that you are dreaming but often can also shape the contents and feel of the dream. In a lucid dream, you are not merely a passive observer – you are a conscious co-creator, walking through a world woven by your own imagination and inner truth.

Lucid dreams are not just wildly entertaining or curious anomalies of the sleeping mind. They can be deeply healing, spiritually expansive and psychologically liberating. Within this state, people have found the courage to face their inner demons, to relive painful memories and transform them, to hold imagined conversations with those who have passed and to explore and encounter unconscious parts of themselves that waking life may keep hidden. A lucid dream can be a rehearsal room, a therapist's couch, a sanctuary and a sky to fly through – limitless, luminous and utterly personal.

Many lucid dreamers describe a growing sense of intimacy with the unconscious. Instead of fearing the unpredictable terrain of the dreamworld, they begin to trust it. The dream becomes a temple rather than a trap. And in this space, they meet guides, archetypes, lost memories and sometimes even glimpses of what feels like the soul's deeper longing.

Liminal states and lucid dreams are intimately connected by one essential thread: awareness within transition. Lucid dreaming often begins in two ways: either from within the dream itself, when you 'wake up' and recognize its dreamlike nature; or immediately from the liminal state, when you drift into sleep while remaining conscious, a practice known as wake-initiated lucid dreaming (WILD).

In this technique, as your body begins to soften into sleep and sleep paralysis gently takes hold, your awareness remains steady, like a flame flickering in the dark. You may begin to calmly witness ephemeral images behind your closed eyes – faces that morph and dissolve, celestial landscapes, shimmering patterns or half-formed scenes. Sounds might arise – snatches of music, voices, even whispers. Sensations can emerge too: a sense of floating, spinning or vibrating, as though your dream body is trying to lift away from the physical one. These are the hallmarks of hypnagogic hallucinations and they are the threshold signs that a lucid dream is beginning to bloom.

With practice, patience and gentleness, you can learn not to startle yourself awake but to instead step softly from the liminal realm into the dreamscape. The key is not to force but to follow and to allow consciousness to flow like a river through the passage into sleep. And then, almost miraculously, you find yourself standing in a dream, fully aware, the dream light around you alive with possibility.

To become conscious in a dream is to realize that the boundaries of self, reality and imagination are far more fluid than we are taught. It is a reminder that the soul has wings and that the night does not only bring rest but revelation.

Techniques to trigger lucid dreams

Lucid dreaming doesn't require special talent, only a commitment to inner exploration, a sense of curiosity and a willingness to gently train your awareness. Like meditation or creativity, lucid dreaming is a practice – one that grows deeper and more rewarding the more you engage with it. Whether you're seeking healing, adventure, spiritual insight or simply a deeper connection to your unconscious, there are tried and tested techniques to help you cross the threshold consciously.

One of the most powerful ways to begin is by weaving reality checks into your waking life. Several times a day, pause and ask yourself: 'Am I dreaming?' Try to push your finger through your palm and if you are dreaming, it will go right through. Observe the details of your surroundings, or glance at a digital clock twice; objects and numbers often behave erratically in dreams. These small acts of questioning encourage a habit of awareness that can carry over into your dreamscape, because what you do during the day filters into your dreams and vice versa. The moment you ask the question inside a dream is often the moment you realize you're dreaming and lucidity begins.

Another powerful technique is mnemonic induction of lucid dreams (MILD). As you lie in bed preparing for sleep, repeat a simple intention, like a mantra: 'Tonight, I will realize I am dreaming.' As you do this, visualize yourself inside a dream, noticing something strange – a floating object, an unusual person, a familiar location made unfamiliar – and becoming lucid. This primes the mind to recognize the dream state from within.

The wake-back-to-bed (WBTB) method is especially effective, but please note it should only be used when you don't need to work, drive, or operate machinery the next day, as it can disrupt sleep. After four to six hours of sleep, when your REM cycles are longest, gently wake yourself. Stay up for 15 to 30 minutes. During this time, read about dreaming, write in your dream journal or meditate. Then return to bed with focused intent. This practice increases the chance of re-entering sleep while maintaining a thread of awareness and it's during this twilight state that lucidity often naturally arises.

Dream journalling is also essential. Keep a notebook or

voice recorder by your bed and upon waking, even in the middle of the night, record every detail you can remember, no matter how fragmented or strange. This strengthens your dream recall and reveals patterns, themes and dream signs unique to your psyche. You may notice a symbol, a particular animal, person or sensation that repeats itself. These doorways to awareness become your personal 'lucidity cues', so when you encounter them again in a dream you can perhaps tell yourself that you are dreaming and become lucid.

With time, patience and care, these techniques can open the gates to a realm where magic, memory and meaning converge. The key is not to force lucidity but to court it so it surfaces naturally and to approach it with the reverence of a seeker and the openness of a child. Lucid dreaming is not about control; it's about connection. Connection to the deepest parts of yourself. Connection to a wisdom that speaks in symbols. Connection to the vast, mysterious intelligence that dreams through and within you. Indeed, I have found that the best way to have a lucid dream naturally is to simply get into the life-changing habit of writing dreams down on waking, reflecting on their meaning during the day and setting the intention to lucid dream just before sleeping.

Yoga Nidra: A Conscious Descent into Sleep

There is an ancient practice that mirrors and magnifies the liminal experience: yoga nidra, or yogic sleep. Far more than simple relaxation, yoga nidra is a sacred art, a conscious descent into sleep where the physical body rests but the inner witness remains awake. Unlike traditional sleep, in which we surrender awareness completely, yoga nidra invites us to soften into a state where the boundaries between waking and dreaming dissolve and the soul becomes luminous in its own stillness.

Practised lying down in a supported, comfortable position, the session begins with a guided audio narration through the landscape of the body, breath, emotions and imagery. You are led gently by a calming voice into a space where the thinking mind begins to quiet, yet awareness hovers just above the threshold of unconsciousness. It is a state akin to deep non-REM rest, a physiological sleep with the lucidity of meditative awareness intact.

In this powerful space, you can witness yourself falling asleep without losing consciousness, an extraordinarily rare experience in modern life. It is the cultivation of the hypnagogic state with intention. Here, the veil thins. You may glimpse dream images, hear fragments of inner dialogue or feel the vast spaciousness of your inner world unfolding.

More than a technique for rest, yoga nidra is a portal to healing. Clinical studies now affirm what the ancient yogis always knew: that this practice can help to ease anxiety, soothe insomnia, reduce symptoms of PTSD and even alleviate chronic pain. It downshifts the nervous system, activates the body's innate capacity for repair and opens the door to profound emotional release. But beyond even these benefits, there is a deeper gift.

Yoga nidra is a practice of self-remembering. It reveals that awareness does not have to vanish with sleep. It teaches us that consciousness is not confined to waking life but is a golden thread that runs through all states of being. In the quiet of yoga nidra, we are reminded of who we are beneath the noise: spacious, grounded and connected to something far greater than the individual self.

To practise yoga nidra is to learn the language of liminality. It is to float gently in that sacred in-between, where healing, dreaming and waking merge. In a world obsessed with doing, yoga nidra offers the radical invitation to just *be* – and in that being, to remember the timeless awareness that watches over us all, even as we sleep.

Dream Incubation

Long before modern psychology, seekers at the temples of Asclepius in Ancient Greece would recline in quiet stone chambers, intentionally inviting the realm of dreams to bring them healing and guidance. This ancient ritual, known as dream incubation, is the art of consciously planting a seed before sleep in the liminal state, setting a focused intention to engage in conversation with the dreaming mind.

This practice has not been lost to time and persists today in various forms, sometimes called dream seeding or dreamscaping. At its heart lies a simple, profound gesture: before drifting into sleep, when you are close to that highly impressionable liminal state, you pose a question to your inner world. It might be a profound enquiry such as, 'What part of myself needs healing?' or a practical concern like, 'How can I navigate this challenge in my life?'

The liminal space between waking and sleeping, the hypnagogic threshold, is crucial here. As you surrender to the gentle pull of sleep, you hold your question lightly, like a feather floating on a still pond. It is in this delicate state that fragments of images, sensations or fleeting scenes often begin to emerge, quietly answering your call. These glimpses may evolve into a full dream or resurface as you awaken, caught in the misty veil of hypnopompia.

Dream incubation reconnects us with an inner oracle – not a supernatural force but a deep, wise intelligence residing in the unconscious. The messages you receive might not come wrapped in words or clear statements; more often, they arrive as symbols, emotions, questions, leaps of faith or vivid fragments of narrative. Yet with patience and attentive listening, patterns form, insights deepen and a quiet knowing takes root.

In this way, dream incubation is more than a technique; it is a nightly sacred dialogue with the soul. It invites us to become co-creators in our own healing and growth, reminding us that the answers we seek are often already present within the quiet depths of our dreaming mind, waiting to be uncovered under the twilight canopy of sleep. In essence, what you tell yourself before you go to sleep may not only change your dreams but your life too.

False Awakenings

Among the most mystifying experiences in the twilight territories of consciousness are false awakenings, moments when you dream that you have woken up, performed your morning rituals, moved through your day, only to truly awaken later and realize that none of it was real. These dreams play tricks on the mind, weaving elaborate layers of waking life that feel startlingly authentic, blurring the lines between sleep and reality.

Sometimes false awakenings arrive in a cascade of nested layers: you awaken, dress, step into your day, then 'wake up' again, each awakening feeling more vivid than the last. In more unsettling instances, people find themselves caught in endless loops, struggling to break free, panic mounting as each attempt to awaken fails. These loops are the mind's way of struggling to reorient itself, a glitch in the transition between sleep and wakefulness.

False awakenings most often occur during those fragile border crossings when the mind is partially alert yet still tethered to REM sleep. It's as if the brain is attempting to reboot while still dreaming, caught between worlds. For those who practise lucid dreaming, these confusing loops can be transformed into moments of empowerment. Recognizing the repetition as a sign you are dreaming can become a key unlocking the cycle and moving you deeper into conscious dreaming.

The true secret to navigating false awakenings is once again to soften your response. Rather than dreading these confusing echoes, understand them as signals, messages from the liminal self. They often arrive when something vital is waiting to be remembered or integrated, a piece of wisdom or a hidden fragment of the psyche lingering on the threshold, inviting your attention.

Losing Fear and Gaining Wonder

So much of modern life teaches us to rush past the edges of consciousness, to flee the blurry, uncertain moments where sleep and wakefulness – the conscious and unconscious – overlap and when you are neither fully awake nor dreaming big. We bolt into full awareness or slip quickly into deep sleep, avoiding any kind of confrontation with the strange fog, the shadowy figures, the sensation of floating outside our bodies. Yet what if those edges, the liminal spaces between worlds, are not places of danger but of profound sacredness?

What if instead of recoiling from hypnagogic visions or paralysing moments, we welcomed them with gentle curiosity? What if, rather than shrinking away in fear, we stood calmly at this border and asked with open hearts, 'What are you here to teach me?'

When we release anxiety about them, these mysterious states help us reclaim some of the most extraordinary gifts of the human psyche: the capacity to imagine without boundaries, to converse with the unconscious, to dream with intention and to witness ourselves undergoing profound transformation from one state of consciousness to another. The edges become a threshold not to be feared but embraced – a liminal library where creativity, wisdom and self-discovery unfold. In this deep space, the boundaries of self soften and the door to infinite possibility both within and all around you swings wide open.

Exercises and Practices for Liminal Exploration

To conclude, here are some accessible yet profoundly effective practices you can start incorporating immediately – simple reminders to step respectfully into the mysterious borderlands between waking and sleeping. Together, these exercises invite you to cultivate a curious, tender relationship with the liminal spaces of sleep.

Train yourself to wake naturally

Alarm clocks are the enemy of dream recall and working with the transformative and creative potential of the liminal states. This is because they shock your mind and body too swiftly into the conscious waking state, making it hard for liminal imagery to stay on your mind.

Waking naturally is something you can learn to do. Before you go to sleep each night, simply set the intention to wake naturally and prove to yourself that you can do it and that your inner world (not your alarm) can set the tone for your day. If you are worried you might oversleep, set the intention to wake up a few minutes before your alarm. You will be surprised how often you can successfully do this, and when you do, let it again be a reminder that you can wake *yourself* up and set the empowered tone for your day and the rest of your life.

Hypnagogic art practice

As you begin to drift towards sleep, pay close attention to the very first images, shapes or colours that float into your awareness. The moment you catch one – pause. Before fully surrendering to sleep, gently rouse yourself just enough to reach for a notebook or sketchpad by your bedside.

Don't worry about creating something polished or logical. The image might be a blurred face, a flash of colour, a fragment of a phrase or an abstract shape. These fleeting impressions are like instant photographs from the edge of the unconscious – raw, honest and rich with meaning. Over days and weeks, you may begin to recognize recurring themes or symbols, which can serve as fertile ground for creative work or self-reflection. Allow these glimpses to inspire writing, music or drawing, or to simply deepen your understanding of your inner landscape.

Similarly, if you find yourself waking up in the early hours of the morning – say between 2am and 5am – don't try to force yourself to go back to sleep or worry that you aren't going to get enough sleep. Sit up and write down whatever is on your mind in your dream journal before settling back down to sleep. Your dreaming mind woke you up for a reason.

It had something very important to tell you. In monasteries, the early hours of the morning when the world is quiet are the sacred call to prayer. Waking in the early hours of the morning is a sacred moment. Treat it as such.

Liminal body awareness

Before sleeping, when you are lying comfortably in bed with your eyes closed, bring your attention inward to your physical self. Without moving, slowly scan your body from the tips of your toes upward to the crown of your head. With each area, silently acknowledge its presence and send love to it: 'I am lovingly aware of my toes . . . I am aware of my feet . . . my ankles . . .' Take your time, savouring each moment of stillness and presence. This mindful body scan calms the nervous system, gently easing anxiety and opening a doorway to hypnagogic awareness. It prepares your mind to hover on the edge of sleep with consciousness intact creating fertile ground for lucid dreaming or simply peaceful rest.

Beginner's yoga nidra practice

Here is a short, simple yoga nidra script you can try on your own. It is designed to guide you gently into a state of deep relaxation while maintaining a thread of mindful awareness:

1. **Set an intention (*sankalpa*).** Lie down in a quiet, comfortable space. Close your eyes and take a few deep, calming breaths. Silently say to yourself: 'I welcome

awareness. I trust the process of rest.' (Or: 'I will remain aware as I fall asleep.')

Your intention is like a planted seed and is something to return to throughout the practice.

2. **Body scan.** Gently bring your loving attention to each part of your body, one at a time. Spend a few seconds noticing sensations without judgement:
right-hand thumb → fingers → palm → wrist → forearm → elbow → upper arm → shoulder. Then move down the right side to toes. Repeat the same sequence on the left side.

   Finish with a slow scan over your head, face, chest, back and abdomen, sensing the rise and fall of your breath.

3. **Breath awareness.** Shift your focus to your breathing. Notice the natural rhythm as the breath flows in and out. Begin counting backwards from ten to one with each exhale – this helps to quiet the mind and deepen relaxation.
4. **Image visualization.** Allow yourself to imagine – or feel, or describe to yourself with your thoughts – one or more of the following peaceful scenes:

   - A slowly turning spiral of light
   - A vast, calm ocean under moonlight
   - A door opening to a softly glowing room
   - A star gently falling through the night sky

Let these images arise naturally and drift away, without forcing or holding onto anything.

5. **Return or release.** When you're ready, choose to either let yourself drift seamlessly into sleep or slowly bring yourself back by counting from one to five. Gently open your eyes, returning to full wakefulness with calm and ease.

For best results, you can record this script, speaking slowly and calmly in your own voice, and play it softly at bedtime or you can find many free yoga nidra scripts to listen to on YouTube. With regular practice, you'll become acquainted with that beautiful paradox yoga nidra offers, where the body sleeps deeply but the mind stays softly aware. It's a doorway into radiant rest, a way to explore the liminal space between wakefulness and sleep with gentle curiosity.

A note on insomnia

For those who suffer from insomnia, the night can feel like an enemy – an endless stretch of time where the mind races, the body resists rest and every passing hour feels like a theft of vitality.

The frustration of trying to force sleep often only deepens the problem. But approaching the night differently through exploration and enjoyment of the liminal states can ease the burden. Instead of wrestling with sleep, we can learn to befriend the in-between. Practices like yoga nidra and dream incubation offer a shift in focus: from demanding unconsciousness to welcoming stillness and subtle inner states for the insight and creativity they can bring. Even if sleep remains elusive, radiant rest becomes possible. And from rest, eventually, comes renewal. The liminal states can be healing companions for the sleepless, soft bridges that invite calm, creativity and eventual surrender, without pressure or judgement.

Dream-incubation ritual

Try this simple method of dream incubation, or dreamscaping:

- Before bed, write a question in your journal or whisper it aloud three times. For example: 'What do I need to understand about my current path?' or 'Is this relationship in my best interests?'
- Lie quietly and repeat the question as you fall asleep, not with effort but with softness – like a sacred invitation. Let it hover at the edge of your thoughts, just as the world begins to blur and your body starts to let go.
- This moment, the in-between, is where the magic happens. It is here, in the hush between wakefulness and dreaming, that the unconscious begins to stir. Your question becomes a thread, weaving its way into the dreamworld.
- When you awaken, stay still. Let the dream linger. What do you remember? A symbol? A person? A scene?

- Write it down, even if it feels fragmented or strange. Dreams speak in images, not explanations. Then, later in the day, brainstorm your dream's meaning.

Repeat this for several nights or make it a nightly ritual. The liminal moment just before sleep is a doorway, fragile, powerful and ancient. Ask with humility and your dreams will answer you in their own language, in their own time.

False-awakening reality check

If you've ever woken up only to realize you were still dreaming, you've encountered the strange mirror of a false awakening. These moments can be disorienting but they are also golden gateways into conscious dreaming. They occur in the liminal zone where waking and dreaming overlap, a threshold space charged with mystery and potential.

To navigate them:

- Perform a reality check each morning: as with the process outlined for lucid dreaming (see page 167), try pushing your finger through your opposite palm or glance at a digital clock twice (in dreams, the numbers often shift). If you do these checks every day, when the mind wavers between realms, they become like anchors and you are more likely to do them in the dream state. But if you do them while you are dreaming, something odd or bizarre will happen that couldn't happen in waking reality. For example, your fingers will push right through your palm or you find yourself with six fingers on one hand.

- If you find yourself in a dream version of your room, pause. Don't rush or panic. Look around and softly ask, 'What am I supposed to notice?' Let the dream speak to you in its language of symbols and shifts.
- Use false awakenings as springboards into dream lucidity. The moment you sense the unreal within the familiar, you are already halfway to becoming fully aware within the dream.

Rather than fearing the repetition or confusion, greet these loops as portals. You are brushing the edges of awareness, dancing along the veil. It's not madness, it's mastery. And every time you wake within a dream, you're remembering that your consciousness is far vaster than the waking world allows.

Daydream believer

Not all liminal states require sleep. Daydreaming also exists in this subtle twilight between intention and surrender, between the logic of waking thought and the openness of the dreaming mind. This is another potential opportunity for extreme dreaming that is easily overlooked in our fast-moving world; yet when approached with awareness, daydreaming becomes a sacred space of creation.

When used intentionally, daydreaming becomes more than idle drifting. It becomes a magnet for manifestation, a rehearsal for the reality you dream about and a way to speak to your unconscious in the language it understands – imagery, feeling, symbol.

Here's how to make it practical:

- Sit quietly for five minutes with your eyes closed. Take a breath and recall something you want to call into your waking life – a feeling, a project, a healing, a connection.
- Instead of thinking in words, let images or feelings rise naturally. See yourself already immersed in that desired reality. Feel it happening in your body.
- Don't analyse or judge. Just let the vision unfold like a soft inner film, shaped by heart more than logic.
- When you're finished, write down what you saw and felt. Even the smallest image holds meaning. Remind yourself that if you can dream it and believe in that dream, you can do it, as the brain does not know the difference between the dreaming and waking state.

This is not escapism. It is energetic alignment. Repeated, focused daydreaming rooted in emotion and imagery activates your nervous system, your motivation and your sense of possibility. It is a liminal tool, ancient and modern, and a way to dream with your eyes wide open. And its power lies not in fantasy but in the quiet way it reorients your unconscious beliefs – because if you can see yourself doing something in either the dreaming or daydreaming state, your mind is more likely to believe it is possible. And when your mind believes something is possible for you, it often is. Like energy seeks like energy. Manifestation 101.

Liminal Living

Every night and every morning, we pass through hypnagogia and hypnopompia, those fragile, mysterious states, often without noticing. But to notice them is to awaken.

Another important reminder that liminal dreaming, sleep paralysis, false awakenings and lucid dreaming are not flaws in the architecture of sleep. They are keys to your inner world, a precious opportunity to reshape your relationship with fear, to brainstorm and make connections and leaps of faith and to reconnect with the creative language of your soul.

They are training grounds for consciousness itself. And the more intimately you explore them, the more you learn to stay grounded – not only in dreams but in your waking life too and in those unpredictable moments of transition when the old has fallen away but the new has not yet arrived. Heartbreak, transformation, birth, loss, sudden clarity, identity shift and so on. These are not detours; they too are thresholds. When you encounter them, let go. Breathe. Witness. You are not lost. You are between. And between is where all the magic lives.

Let this chapter teach you how to walk through the liminal mist with your eyes, mind and heart wide open from now on. To stand in the doorway and greet whatever shadows and opportunities for growth await you there. Because just beyond the edge of dreaming, something deeper waits. Not darkness but depth. Not an ending but an invisible thread pulling you towards a higher and wiser version of yourself.

In the next chapter, we follow that thread to its natural destination and inspiration – into those dreams that dare to speak of death and what on earth or in heaven they might be trying to awaken in us.

5

DEADLY DREAMING

It starts with the wind: sharp, sudden, impossible to brace against. One moment you're standing on solid ground, high above everything and the next, that ground vanishes beneath your feet. You're falling. Not slipping. Not stumbling. Falling, fast, helpless, headlong through empty space. The sky above spins away as the earth below rushes up like a threat. There is no control, no time to think, only the hollow scream trapped in your throat and the sickening lurch of your stomach as gravity takes everything. The dream makes it feel endless. Seconds stretch into lifetimes. You see flashes as you fall, your hands reaching, grasping at nothing, the blur of trees or towers or jagged cliff-face spinning past, too fast to hold onto. Your mind scrambles for logic, for escape but deep down you know: this isn't just a fall; this is the end.

The dream has become a descent into death itself. You can feel it. The air grows colder, thinner, as though the world is letting go of you before you even hit the ground. Time warps. Fear sharpens. And then, just before impact, everything slows. You see the earth waiting to catch you like a closed fist. You feel your body brace, heart pounding once, then twice. And then nothing. The dream doesn't show the moment of death. It doesn't need to. The silence says it all. You don't wake. You hang there in the void, suspended between the breath you didn't finish and the one you'll never take. The fall becomes a metaphor your soul already understands – that dying is not just an end but a letting go so complete that even the dream must release you. And in that final moment, as blackness takes your place, you realize – it wasn't the fall in the dream that terrified you. It was the silence waiting at the bottom . . .

Falling in a dream – plummeting helplessly through the air into the unknown, gravity pulling you towards what feels like certain death – is consistently reported as the most common dream theme across cultures, age groups and generations. When researchers compile lists of the hundred most frequently reported dreams worldwide, the sensation of falling usually ending just before impact always rises to the top. Or rather, drops.

Why is falling a near-universal dream theme?

Because it taps into something ancient and primal: the instinctive terror of losing control, of being ripped away from solid ground and the dreadful certainty that something has gone terribly wrong. At its core, falling symbolizes our deepest anxieties – those moments in life when the foundation beneath us vanishes emotionally, spiritually or existentially.

It's no coincidence that death hovers at the edges of these dreams. The Grim Reaper – symbol of the unknown, of endings – is never far away in them. In our sleeping minds, death waits at the bottom, unseen but undeniably felt. A reminder that mortality is always just beneath the surface of our most vulnerable states.

A few years ago, I had such a dream at a time when my life was slipping out from under me. It came shortly after my husband was diagnosed with Alzheimer's. The days were heavy with confusion and panic. The nights full of questions I couldn't answer. And slowly my dreams began to speak for me and bring their healing.

Dream journal entry – 12 April 2018

> Someone is standing alone on the edge of a crumbling cliff. Below, there is nothing but blackness – vast, silent, endless. They don't jump. The ground simply disappears beneath them.
>
> There's no scream. No struggle. Just a long, slow descent. A quiet fall into the void. Time stretches and bends. Just as the crash seems inevitable, something

> shifts. They are no longer falling, but floating suspended in dark water that feels strangely warm.

That dream, more than any doctor's words or well-meaning advice, helped me begin to understand what was happening. The fall symbolism represented coming death – not literal death but the death of certainty, of stability, of the life my husband and I had planned together. It was the symbolic death of the versions of me and of him that I had always known. And yet, like most falling dreams, this dream didn't end in destruction. Usually, when you are falling in a dream you wake up before you land, and my dream fall shapeshifted into floating. Although the water I was suspended in was dark, it felt warm. This showed me that even in the face of profound loss, something comforting and hopeful would remain.

In dreaming of falling, I unknowingly began to grieve but I also began to accept and heal. Remember, dreams often tell us the truths we can't yet face in waking life. That night, mine told me this: I was falling, for sure. My life had changed forever. But within me was a buoyancy I hadn't yet discovered and that has continued to keep me afloat.

Dying to Live

We do not dream of death and dying because we want to die. We dream of death because we feel uncertain and helpless and long to live fully – and because somewhere deep inside, we know that we are not and that we need to find new ways to not just survive but thrive.

The death of ourselves or someone else is another near-universal nightmare theme, consistently reported across time, culture and age. Often, as discussed above, we are falling endlessly and just before we hit the ground . . . the sensation of blackness and our own impending doom. Sometimes, we are being chased by a faceless murderer, a car veers off the road, the plane begins to shake, the waves pull us under. Perhaps we are in hospital beds or graveyards, witnessing our own funerals, seeing people who know and love us weep, forget to attend or celebrate. And sometimes, the death theme is not centre stage but waiting in the wings: a terminal diagnosis, a withering body, an unexplained shadow looming on the horizon. Or we find ourselves watching loved ones die in our dreams, sometimes at our own hands. Our dreams transforming us overnight into murderers.

There is a disorienting quality to these deadly dreams that makes them hard to shake. Even if we wake and realize we and those we love are alive and well, our nervous systems take a while to adjust. The breath is shallow, the heart races and the body remains locked in a low-grade panic. Sometimes the feeling of grief and loss for our own dream death or the dream death of others may irrationally haunt us for hours or linger on with us for days.

We often assume that to dream of death is a premonition, a message from the unconscious that something terrible is about to happen. And in some rare cases, death dreams do correspond with real events, suggesting a kind of intuitive foreshadowing, which we will discuss in Chapter Six. But in most cases these dreams are symbolic, not literal. They are the mind's desperate attempt to get our attention because it has learned that of all the countless metaphors it can send us death is the one that never fails to get our attention.

The Symbolism of Death in Dreams

Death in dreams is rarely about dying. It is typically about the inevitability of change, the only constant in life. About endings. About the crumbling of old selves, old beliefs, old lives. And it's about our resistance to letting go.

In most psychological and spiritual traditions, death is not the end but rather a transformation, the darkness before the dawn. To die in a dream may indicate that some part of us is being called to evolve, or to surrender and release its grip over us. Perhaps a version of yourself that no longer serves you is ready to be laid to rest: the perfectionist, the people-pleaser, the codependent, the exhausted over-achiever.

Dreaming of your own death can be disturbing. But when interpreted symbolically, it often signals the arrival of a new self that is waiting to be born. It's the psyche's way of saying: 'This way of being is finished. It has taught you all it can. Time now to let it go.'

Dreams of others dying – friends, family, strangers – can reflect our emotional distance from them, our fear of losing them or parts of ourselves we associate with them. A parent dying in a dream might not be about literal loss but about growing up. A child's death could represent the end of innocence or the pressures of responsibility. And being murdered, attacked or executed often speaks to feeling that you are a victim of forces beyond your control. What part of yourself is under attack? What beliefs or emotions are you trying to kill off or are being threatened by others?

Seen through this lens, death in dreams is less about disaster and more about identity. Who are you now? Who are you becoming? And what mindsets, relationships or situations must you release to get there?

When Death Dreams Reflect Trauma

While symbolic interpretation is vital, we must also acknowledge that some death dreams are trauma dreams. When life becomes overwhelming through grief, abuse, burnout, illness or heartbreak, our unconscious doesn't respond with gentle metaphors. It responds with alarm bells.

If you've lived through trauma, or experienced high stress, you may have had extremely disturbing dreams with the following themes: falling from great heights, drowning or suffocating, being stabbed, murdered, executed or shot, being chased and caught, seeing your own corpse or a loved one's.

These nightmares don't arrive to scare you. They arrive

because your mind is attempting to cathartically process what it cannot make sense of during the day. They are the emotional residue of terror, stored in the nervous system and replayed in symbols at night. Trauma lives in the body. When we are in survival mode, our waking mind may deny or minimize pain just to keep functioning. But dreams do not lie. They reveal, in sometimes terrifying clarity, the unfelt feelings. The threat may be over but the body doesn't yet know that. It needs time to process everything and it will do that through extreme dreams. Give it that time and feel gratitude for the deep healing your dreaming mind is doing on your behalf.

These nightmares are the psyche's way of making sense of things. And when we begin to listen – without fear, without judgement – and understand what is triggering them, we can begin to heal.

Death as the Ultimate Archetype

To understand why death so often appears in dreams, we must face a deeper truth: death is the final archetype, the deepest and darkest and most unknown shadow in the human mind. Not because it is evil or malicious but because it is inescapable.

In Jungian psychology, archetypes are patterns of meaning, primordial images and energies that live deep in the collective unconscious – in other words, common to us all. The 'Mother', the 'Warrior', the 'Lover', the 'Shadow'.

And among them, the 'Death' archetype stands supreme not as a destroyer but as an opportunity to be reborn.

To dream of death is to confront the edge of identity. To face what we are clinging to. And usually what we fear in death is not oblivion but emptiness. We are terrified that our lives will not have mattered. That our connections will dissolve. That the self we've worked so hard to build will vanish like fog. But beneath this often lies a deeper fear: the fear of living fully.

Paradoxically, when people say they are afraid of death, what they often mean is that they are afraid of life not lived. The missed chances. The silence where their voice should be. The dreams left unloved. The self that is left unexpressed.

In this way, death dreams are the most serious wakeup calls. They are not warnings that you will die tomorrow but invitations to ask: 'Am I alive today?' It's easy to numb ourselves when life feels confusing. To follow familiar routines, stick to the same mindset, to live or bury our desires under responsibility. But the unconscious knows better. It will not let you sleepwalk through your own life. It will send you the symbolism of death – chilling, faceless, often violent – not as a punishment but as a jolt into your dreams. A shakedown of your inner world. A call to courage and to step outside your comfort zone more often in your waking life.

The Psychology of the Death Wish

In some cases, death dreams come from an even deeper, darker place, which is not fear of death but instead an irrational pull towards it. This is what Freud termed the 'death drive', or Thanatos, a force within the psyche that seeks rest, silence, dissolution, nothingness. It is the counterpart to Eros, the drive towards life, creation and desire.

In dreams, this longing may appear as scenarios of wishing to vanish or melt away, being invisible, walking into the sea and not turning back, lying down in a grave peacefully and embracing death as a friend. And sometimes dreams of having sex can be a metaphor for the death wish. Freud linked the death wish to sex by suggesting that the two instincts are intertwined. Even in erotic or steamy dreams, the pull towards surrender, loss of control or merging with another can symbolically express a longing for the ultimate release: a return to nothingness.

Both death-themed and intensely erotic dreams can be deeply unsettling. But they also have meaning. They tell us that a part of us is deeply tired. Worn out by life's demands. Longing for peace and escape. These are dreams that must be held gently; they should be interpreted with compassion, not alarm or shame. They point to an urgent need for change, for letting go of something unbearable or unsustainable. A relationship. A job. A role. A mask. They become a metaphor not of a desire to end life but for ending the suffering caused by a mindset, situation or relationship that is draining your life force. And if the suffering can't be ended, then the dream is seeking to find a way to transform it into purpose.

Recurring Death Dreams: When the Soul Insists

It is one thing to dream of death and/or sex once. It is another to dream of it night after night. Some dreams do not simply pass. They return, repeatedly. Whether the theme is death, falling, being chased, teeth crumbling or apocalypse, recurring nightmares are often a sign of deeply unresolved internal conflict or fear.

When an extreme dream repeats it may signal a traumatic memory or unresolved grief, or it could be a lesson not yet learned, a pattern unexamined. The deadly symbols return to shock you into noticing them. Try to reflect on when the recurring nightmare began – that is why keeping a dream journal is key – as painful memories can lie dormant for years and then be triggered by events in your waking life that remind you of the original trauma.

People experiencing major life transitions – divorce, career change, grief, trauma recovery – often report persistent death dreams. Sometimes the dreams stop only when the dreamer makes a real-life change – ends a toxic relationship, starts therapy or begins to express something they have long suppressed. Recurring nightmares are a message: something must die so there is space for something else, something better to move in and live. They are the soul's way of insisting: 'You cannot stay here. You have outstayed your welcome.'

Recurring death dreams or intense nightmares emerge when we are ignoring something vital or holding onto mindsets, people or things that we have outgrown or expectations of others that no longer match our own. The unconscious is patient but not endlessly so. If a truth is being avoided in waking life, it will knock at the door first in your dreams. If it is ignored there too, it will eventually pound. If it is still denied, it may enter your waking life uninvited, in intrusive thoughts.

Recurring dreams are not a malfunction; they are a form of persistent self-help. The psyche does not give up on what matters. Just as physical wounds keep bleeding until they are treated, psychic wounds reappear in dreams until they are witnessed and integrated. The goal is not to eliminate the dream but to change your relationship with it. Often, when you approach the recurring nightmare with fascination rather than avoidance and understand what it is trying to teach you, it softens or transforms entirely.

How Waking Fears Create Death Dreams

As we have explored, dreams are deeply intelligent responses to our inner and outer environment. When we are carrying anxiety, fear or unprocessed emotions during the day, they do not vanish at bedtime. Instead, they follow us into the darkness, shapeshifting into metaphor, narrative and image. This is particularly true of death-themed dreams. When we are overwhelmed by real-life transitions such as job instability, illness, emotional isolation or relationship uncertainty, the unconscious responds by constructing imagery that mirrors the magnitude of our stress. And what could feel more definitive, more absolute, than death?

Death dreams often emerge when we feel trapped or out of control in waking life. Our sense of aliveness is being threatened not by literal death but by emotional suffocation, stagnation or existential despair. The dream then says: 'This life as you know it just cannot continue.' And because the unconscious doesn't speak in polite conversation, it dramatizes this truth using its most powerful symbol: death.

It's easy to feel betrayed by repeating dreams, as though they're designed to freak you out, but more often they are internal emergency broadcasts: your inner world needs attention. You are not fine. And they'll keep coming back for you time and time again until you listen to what they want you to know and make a change.

Intense Dreams as Stress Release and Solution-Seekers

As scary as some dreams may be, it is healing to know that even the most intense nightmares have a message and a function. The dreaming brain – especially during REM – attempts to process, release and even resolve difficult emotional material we haven't consciously worked through. Nightmares metabolize stress and help you move towards healing. Think of them in the same way you might think of a fever as an encouraging sign that the body is trying to expel toxins.

Intense dreams can also be compared to emotional compression chambers. They squeeze the energy that's been building in your system and try to reorganize it, however clumsily, into meaning, expression and action. Every nightmare of death, murder, porn or shocking violence can be helping us to express what we repress in waking life, nudging us to face the reality of endings we're avoiding, preparing us for emotional shifts we're resisting, rehearsing responses to fear in a safe environment or revealing internal parts of ourselves that are in need of integration. In other words, dreams – especially deadly and disturbing dreams – are always trying to restore inner balance. They are like psychological pressure valves. They won't always be pretty, but they are always purposeful.

When Death Dreams Come for Loved Ones

Few dreams are as distressing as those in which a loved one dies. Whether the dream is graphic, quiet, symbolic or surreal, the emotional impact can feel devastating, even if we know upon waking that the person is fine. So why do we dream about others dying?

These dreams rarely mean that someone we care about is at risk of dying. Instead, they often reflect shifts in your relationship or within yourself. For example, dreaming of a parent dying may reflect your own maturing or emotional separation from them; dreams of a partner dying may indicate emotional distance, unspoken fears or transformation within the relationship; and dreams of a child dying can symbolize your own loss of innocence or your fear of failing them.

Sometimes, death dreams about loved ones occur when we are pulling away from someone emotionally, consciously or not. The dream acts as a metaphor for the ending of an attachment or our fear of such an ending. Many parents, for example, dream of their adult child dying in a car crash when their child moves out or goes to university. The dreaming mind is trying to help the parent understand that the relationship between parent and child needs to evolve.

Other times, the dream is a wakeup call: a reminder of our own impermanence, of unspoken love or of the need to reconnect with what makes us feel passionate in our waking lives before it's too late. In any of these cases, the dream is never about death itself. It's about the urgency of living with more presence, more intention and more truth, especially with the people we love.

Elena and Mateo: meeting their dream reapers

Elena told me about a recurring dream she'd had every few months for two years.

'I'm in a dark forest,' she said. 'I'm running. I know something is chasing me, but I can't see it. I fall into a shallow grave and dirt starts pouring over me. I scream, but no sound

comes out. Just before I suffocate, I wake up shaking and crying.'

She was convinced this was a premonition of her own death.

But when we explored the dream's context, a deeper story emerged. Around the time the dream began, she had started suppressing her writing. Fear of failure, fear of judgement and the pressure to be successful had paralysed her. The dream wasn't about dying. It was about being buried alive by silence, by fear, by self-criticism.

In working with the dream, she began journalling again. Then writing short stories. Eventually, she self-published a memoir. The dream stopped. And when it returned once more – five years later – it had changed. This time, she rose from the grave, brushed the dirt from her skin and walked out of the forest into sunlight.

Mateo was shaken by a recurring dream he'd been having on and off for over a year. He told me: 'In the dream, my partner is lying in a hospital bed. I'm holding his hand, but I can feel him slipping away. The machines start beeping, the room fills with light and I scream for someone to help. No one comes. His eyes close and I wake up gasping, heart racing, drenched in sweat.' Mateo was terrified this dream meant something was going to happen to his partner; that it was a warning he couldn't ignore.

But, as with Elena, a more personal truth emerged when we explored the dream's context. Around the time the dream began, Mateo's partner had been offered a job abroad. Mateo had supported him but, deep down, he feared being left behind, emotionally and physically. The dream wasn't predicting his death. It was expressing his unspoken grief over the changes in their relationship – the loss of closeness, the fear of growing apart.

As he worked through these feelings, he began to open more to his partner. They had hard, honest conversations. They made time for each other in new ways.

The dream eased. And when it returned, a month later, it had changed. This time, Mateo's partner still lay in the hospital bed but when Mateo reached for his hand, he opened his eyes and smiled. The beeping stopped. The light faded. They were still there, together. And Mateo woke up in tears, but this time from relief.

The Language of Death in Dreams

To recap: the most common symbol for transformation is death and death in dreams is almost always a metaphor for the need for change in your waking life. We dream of crashing cars, terminal illness, funerals or violent ends not because we or someone we love are physically dying but because something needs to end – an identity, a belief, a phase of life, a relationship or an illusion of safety – so something new can take its place.

When we learn to speak the language of metaphor, death dreams become not alarming omens but meaningful symbols of transition to new beginnings. They ask questions such as: 'What needs to end in your life or in a relationship or situation?' 'What are you afraid of releasing?' 'What new self is waiting to be born?'

Don't get too comfortable, though. Dreams are by nature mysterious and elusive and refuse to fall into neat categories. Like the ocean, you can learn to navigate the world of the dream, but you can never fully control or understand its infinite mystery. In extremely rare cases, dreams can predict alarming outcomes in your waking life or in the waking lives of others. These kinds of literal or precognitive or 'psychic' dreams which may – and I stress *may* – be a warning have a very different feel to symbolic or psychological dreams and will be discussed in the next chapter.

Dreaming the Dead

Night visions of departed loved ones also do not fit neatly into the symbolic. According to a recent survey by the Pew Research Center, around half of US adults have dreamed of departed loved ones.* These kinds of afterlife dreams

* Patricia Tevington and Manolo Corichi, 'Many Americans Report Interacting with Dead Relatives in Dreams or Other Ways', Pew Research Center, 23 August 2023, <https://www.pewresearch.org/short-reads/2023/08/23/many-americans-report-interacting-with-dead-relatives-in-dreams-or-other-ways/> [accessed 20 November 2025].

typically happen soon after their death but can also occur years later and are more common than you think. Research from the University of Northampton's parapsychology department suggests that such dreams can help people process grief.* This is in keeping with research suggesting that lucid dreamwork can help ease the pain and distress experienced by veterans suffering from PTSD.† Whether they are afterlife signs or visitations depends on your beliefs regarding afterlife, but whatever they are, for those who dream them they are a loving reminder that death ends a life and not a relationship.

This is not the place to debate the existence of an afterlife, but there is growing research exploring its potential existence just as there is into the healing power of the dreaming mind. A review of the literature indicates that in recent decades there has been a dramatic increase in the number of reported near-death experience (NDE) stories, where people 'died' and were brought back to life and report glimpses of heaven or the 'other side'.‡ This increase is thanks to the miracle of modern

* Calvin E Cooper, 'Spontaneous Post-Death Experiences and the Cognition of Hope: An Examination of Bereavement and Recovery' (unpublished doctoral thesis, University of Northampton, 2017).

† Garret Yount et al., 'Decreased Posttraumatic Stress Disorder Symptoms Following a Lucid Dream Healing Workshop', *Traumatology*, 30(4) (2024), pp. 550–558, doi: 10.1037/trm0000456.

‡ Sandra Barreto, 'Near-Death Experiences: A Bibliometric and Systematic Review of Published Literature From 1977 to 2025', *OMEGA – Journal of Death and Dying*, 0(0) (2025), doi: 10.1177/00302228251363788.

resuscitation techniques – in past times, many of these people would have died and taken their golden stories with them.

According to some quantitative research, many NDE stories share striking similarities.* For instance, NDEs typically involve leaving the body and floating towards a bright light, and they suggest that your learning and evolution does not end when you die and that you get to reconnect with departed loved ones and pets as well as angels and spirit guides. You no longer have a body, but you know that unconditional love and spiritual evolution are the meaning of your life. You can hear the prayers of those left behind.

Mediums say that departed loved ones often choose to meet us in our dreams because it is the easiest way for them to do so and the way that is least likely to cause alarm to the dreamer. There is no proof of an afterlife as such, but the countless messages and experiences people have shared with me for close to three decades indicate that people who experience afterlife dreams often find them deeply reassuring and that a hallmark of afterlife dreams is that they feel surprisingly realistic. You wake up not in shock and fear or with questions running through your mind, as is typical with extreme symbolic dreams, but instead with a calm

* Charlotte Martial et al., 'The Near-Death Experience Content (NDE-C) scale: Development and Psychometric Validation', *Consciousness and Cognition*, 86 (2020), pp. 1,053–8,100, doi: 10.1016/j.concog.2020.103049.

knowing that death ends a life – not a relationship. You can be comforted by the fact that real love does not know death.

Practices to Befriend Your Deadly Dreams

In the section below, you will find some tools you can use to work with death dreams, recurring nightmares and other unsettling imagery.

Pre-sleep dream programming

Before bed, speak directly to your dreaming mind. Say: 'Tonight, I am safe. I welcome healing dreams. I allow whatever needs to be shown, to be shown gently.'

Write this in your journal or whisper it aloud as you fall asleep. You're training your brain to approach the dreamscape differently, with cooperation rather than fear.

Gentle daytime rehearsal

If you have a recurring dying-themed nightmare, imagine the dream in daylight, eyes open. See, feel or write down the moment of terror and then imagine responding differently. Speak. Move. Choose.

This practice is called dream rescripting and, as already mentioned, it is successfully used in trauma therapy to reduce nightmare recurrence. It is reminding you once again that your extreme dreams don't happen *to* you. They are created by you, for you and are all about your mindset and what it is attracting into your waking life.

Dream re-entry

Upon waking from a death dream, lie still and re-enter the dream in your mind's eye or with your thoughts. What would you say to death if you could speak to it and it could speak to you?

This is not fantasy. It is active imagination, a dream-dialogue technique that allows unconscious material to be processed with conscious attention. Give it a try. It is surprisingly therapeutic.

Write the dream as a short story. Give death a name – Joe Black, perhaps. Give it a voice. Let it speak to you. Ask: 'What does this deadly dream want me to know?' Sometimes answers emerge from writing that the waking mind couldn't access directly.

Mindset-shifting

Your dreamlife is shaped by your waking thoughts. If you spend your days in self-criticism, hopelessness or repression, your dreams will reflect that, which increases the likelihood of deadly-dream symbolism by night.

Counter this by practising personal-growth tools such as positive affirmations, creativity (journalling, art, reading), honest emotional expression (therapy, conversation) and reflecting on everyday things you are grateful for as you drift off to sleep.

Healing dreams begin with healing thoughts and there is no greater emotional healer than gratitude.

Nighttime body-safety practice

Not all nightmares are purely emotional or psychological. Sometimes, they are the body's way of crying out through symbols, metaphors or even direct sensations. Long before illness shows up in tests or pain becomes chronic, the subconscious may begin to whisper or shout to you first through the dreamworld.

Dreams that include bleeding, broken bones, suffocation, paralysis or being trapped inside a failing body can sometimes parallel real-world physical conditions. Recurring dreams of choking, for instance, might mirror untreated sleep disorders. Being unable to run or move may echo restless legs, autoimmune flareups or chronic fatigue. Even persistent dreams of being invaded or eaten alive have been reported by those later diagnosed with infections, cancer or digestive disorders.

This doesn't mean every disturbing dream is a medical warning. Most are emotional metaphors. But when a dream persists, especially when accompanied by a bodily sensation upon waking, it's wise to pay attention. Your dream may be alerting you to an imbalance in the system, nudging you towards care, testing or simply deeper awareness. A reminder of an important dream-analysis hack here: it is always worth ruling out the possibility of literal interpretation before moving to the symbolic. For example, if you are repeatedly dreaming about your legs cramping do you need a medical checkup to see if there's a problem?

The body has its own language. And in dreams, that language finally gets a voice. To help you listen calmly to this voice before bed, this practice focuses on your heart and belly – the two intuitive centres in your body because of their rich neural connections with the brain. The belly, or gut, contains the enteric nervous system, often called the 'second brain', which has about 100 million neurons that communicate directly with the brain via influencing emotions and decision-making. Similarly, the heart sends signals to the brain through complex neural pathways that affect emotional processing and stress responses. These bidirectional neural connections allow the heart and gut to play key roles in our intuitive feelings and bodily awareness.

Place your left hand on your heart and your right hand on your belly. Breathe slowly and say: 'I am grounded. I am safe. I will return from the dreamworld with whatever I need for my personal growth and holistic wellbeing.'

Simple as it seems, this somatic cue tells your nervous system that you are in tune with it and in touch with your body and your dreams.

Putting death to sleep

In short, dreams about death arise not only when something within us is ending or dying but also when something new is within you and trying to be born. One door must close now before another can open.

When it comes to dreams about the afterlife, they indicate that your current belief – that you are a human being having a spiritual experience – needs to 'pass away'. This allows it to be replaced by a deep understanding that you are a dreaming being having a human experience and that love goes on.

Whether you dream of your own death, the death of others or the ending of a chapter you can't yet identify, remember this: your dreaming mind is not the executioner. It is your inner healer and wisest guide. It will never stop working to lull you into sleep and, once you are there, to wake you up to the awesome medicine of your own inner wisdom.

6

THE FUTURE OF 'BAD' DREAMS

In this chapter you will see that the future of dreamwork is truly in your own head and hands, along with how you choose to respond to the mind- and heart-opening insights shared in this book. We have come, culturally, to see 'bad dreams' as problems in the psyche. Warnings. Disruptions. Malfunctions. But hopefully you now feel encouraged to radically alter your thinking about all those 'bad' dreams and to start thinking of them like medicine: bitter at first, yes, but ultimately healing.

And to truly appreciate the healing potential of extreme dreams, it is helpful to know how they might evolve through your life, why they come, how to respond and how to distinguish between those that are symbolic and those that are potential, psychic or literal warnings. Each nocturnal journey carries its own message. Each, when welcomed, has the power to transform the dreamer from the inside out.

In recent years, various institutions and individuals have conducted research on how nocturnal dreams change across the human lifespan. For instance, studies on dream-recall frequency and content have been carried out by the Central Institute of Mental Health in Mannheim, Germany, and other research has looked at the emotional content of dreams in adults of different ages.* Collectively, this research evidence contributes to our understanding of how dreams evolve from childhood through to adulthood.

Bad dreams are not random. They shift in tone, content and urgency depending on where we are in our lives. Though every dream is unique, there are patterns and archetypal fears that are likely to emerge at key developmental stages, reflecting our current stage of psychological and emotional growth. Let's begin at the beginning – with the dreams of young children.

Childhood: The Monster Under the Bed

Children's nightmares are often vivid, visceral and overwhelmingly emotional. They can't yet separate dream from reality, so when they dream of being abandoned, eaten, chased or swallowed by darkness, it feels like it really happened.

---

* Marco Zanasi et al., 'Dreams and Age', *Perception and Motor Skills,* 100(3/2) (2005), pp. 925–38, doi: 10.2466/pms.100.3c.925-938.

Common childhood nightmare themes include monsters, wolves, witches, being lost or left behind by parents, falling or drowning, being chased by shadowy figures. One of the most frequently reported recurring dreams for young children is the presence of something scary in their bedroom, like a monster under their bed. Just as with adults, children's bad dreams are often the product of the child feeling they lack control over their circumstances – and 'monsters' represent the scary side of adults when their moods switch. Dreaming of wild-animal attacks can often begin when children start school, reflecting a specific personal or situation there that may be making them feel anxious – a demanding teacher perhaps or a friend rejecting them.

Then there are the commonly reported childhood dreams of ordinary objects – a favoured toy or a household appliance and so on – suddenly becoming menacing. These often occur when there are changes to a child's familiar routine. Such dreams typically reflect the child's growing awareness of separation, mortality and the constant unpredictability of the adult world. A clown at the window might represent a teacher they fear, for instance, or a new sibling stealing attention. The symbolism is direct but powerful.

As children near their teenage years, their dreams start to adjust and reflect their inner struggle with the rules and obligations of the adult world. That is when drowning dreams tend to first appear. Sometimes children dream of discovering an ability to breathe underwater, suggesting the emergence of hidden strengths during times of restriction. Flying dreams and suddenly manifesting unexpected superhero powers can also represent children's desire to soar and discover their own talents. These dreams can feel liberating in contrast to the horrific dreams often reported by older children of being forced to do grisly tasks, such as burying bodies or sorting body parts – sometimes at the command of zombies or abominations. If a child reports this dream, it's a sign they may be feeling pressured to achieve and meet expected standards in their waking life and this is creating within them an ugly fear of not pleasing others or fitting in.

Helping children deal with nightmares

One of the simplest, most powerful things a parent or caregiver can say to a child waking from a nightmare is: 'It felt real, didn't it? Let's talk about it.'

This honours the child's emotional truth, while gently guiding them to not repress or hide what scares them. Never dismiss a child's nightmare; to them, it was real. Then go one step further. Ask them to rescript the dream: 'What would you like to have happened instead?' 'What could your dream-self do differently next time?'

Guide them to imagine they have a sword, a shield, a superhero friend. Let them create an ending where this time they win, escape, fly, laugh. This teaches young people that dreams are not prisons and can be playgrounds for power and creativity – and that the child has far more control over what happens within them than they think. This practice instils emotional regulation, trust in the power of imagination and self-belief – the foundations of a happy dream and waking life.

Teenage Nightmares: Identity and Insecurity

Teenagers face an internal storm in their waking and dreaming lives: hormonal, social, emotional. Dreams at this stage reflect emerging 'adult' fears – rejection, performance anxiety, peer judgement and sexual awakening.

Typical adolescent nightmares may involve scenarios such as public humiliation or nakedness, failing exams, being trapped or feeling powerless and physical transformations such as distorted faces and losing teeth. These reflect the adolescent's fight for autonomy, fear of not being enough and the tension between belonging and becoming.

The classic dream of burying a dead body and not remembering where it is or why you have murdered someone can first appear during this life stage and is directly connected to the need for acceptance and killing aspects of themselves that are deemed unacceptable by others. Dreaming of meeting a celebrity suggests a desire to be noticed and to be admired and dreams about sex are simply curiosity. Dreams about parents and loved ones dying reflect their changing relationship with their parents and their instinctive awareness that their childhood is slipping away.

Adult Nightmares: Pressure and Performance

By adulthood, nightmares commonly shift to reflect themes of emotional suppression and fear of not fitting in and failure. The mood is often frustrating and frenetic. These are no longer dragons in the woods – they're missed flights, losing children or loved ones, natural disasters, infidelity, existential dread. Common adult nightmares also include home invasion, being chased or attacked – often with no visible attacker – witnessing global catastrophe, mistakes in timing or not having the right ID or losing a ticket.

These dreams usually symbolize a disconnection from inner needs. We're too busy. Too responsible. Too exhausted. They arrive like emotional auditors, revealing where we're overextended, disconnected or carrying unresolved guilt and fear, or desperately – and to your own detriment – trying to live up to the expectations of others.

Midlife Nightmares: Mortality and Meaning

In midlife, the unconscious begins to whisper of legacy, mortality and authenticity. Nightmares shift towards endings symbolizing lost youth, broken relationships. Common themes include sudden ageing or death, an unexpected pregnancy or forgotten baby, a house on fire, an abandoned or screaming animal or child.

These are crisis dreams not because something is wrong but because something new wants to be born. The soul wants to be re-evaluated and for the dreamer to reconnect with abandoned parts of themselves and to make more time for themselves and their personal growth. Midlife dreams often signal the death of the false self and the rebirth of purpose.

Dreams of being back at school and not knowing the combination to your locker, having an affair, meeting an ex or searching for something you have lost are urging the dreamer to look back at promises made to themselves that have not been fulfilled or talents that have not yet been expressed. Frustrating dreams involving vehicles, especially out-of-control cars, point to serious career or work challenges and the dreamer's fear of missing out on chances to assert themselves or reveal their talents.

Senior Nightmares: Legacy and the Unknown

As we age into elderhood, dreams can become both more spiritual and more psychic or literal. Nightmares in this phase can feature symbols of death, memory loss, loss of identity. Perhaps the most common later-life dream is the lost purse, phone, bag or wallet – all classic dreams that reflect a sense of disorientation as the world moves faster and becomes less familiar. A dream of being lost in a strange neighbourhood or city, unable to find your way home and with people giving you the wrong directions, is urging the dreamer to make decisions based on what is right for them and not what is convenient for others.

But dreams at this life stage can also be gentle, reflecting a longing for connection, integration and peace. These dreams often bring with them a mystical atmosphere. They are rarely about fear now. More often, they are about acceptance, reconciliation and preparing for a transition – not necessarily death but into a different stage of soul awareness. Many people find their dreams become more intense and memorable in the later years of life, although nightmares may increase because of health issues or shifts in sleeping patterns and medication.

Curiously, people nearing the end of their lives often report that their waking life takes on the quality of a dream itself. Perhaps this is because the world of the dream is who we truly are and those close to passing are reconnecting with their soul, being gently prepared for their next great adventure, their true home.

Gendered Differences

While recurring dream themes of rejection, blood and gore and life and death struggles can happen at any age because they are often linked to stressful conditions and life passages, it is important to bear in mind that their interpretation will be influenced by the stage of life you are in. You always need to look at your waking life to unlock the secret meaning behind your dreams. Gender is another factor to consider as you move forward in your dreamwork.

Every dreamer is unique but tentative research and anecdotal patterns suggest that men and women may dream differently largely because they are socialized to process emotions in different ways.* This is a generalization, of course, but women's nightmares tend to be more interpersonal and emotionally intense, often involving relationship breakdowns or themes of embarrassment and body shame, abandonment, loss of control, babies and children and betrayal by friends. There is also a focus on clothing.

Men's nightmares, by contrast, often reflect themes of violence, physical threat, aggression, being chased or attacked, feeling out of control, sex and failing to protect someone. Weapons feature more strongly in the dreams of men.

This isn't about anything biologically innate; it's about emotional permission. Men are often discouraged from expressing vulnerability in waking life, so their dreams may compensate through symbols of violence or threat. Women are meanwhile conditioned towards emotional caretaking and often process relational traumas and boundary violations in their dreams.

---

* Jonas Mathes and Michael Schredl, 'Gender Differences in Dream Content: Are They Related to Personality?', *International Journal of Dream Research*, 6(2) (2013), pp. 104–109, doi: 10.11588/ijodr.2013.2.10954.

Psychic Dreams: A Different Texture

As foreshadowed in the previous chapter, not all nightmares are symbolic. Some rare ones stand apart from the rest in that they are quieter, sharper, with a clarity that's difficult to explain. These are the psychic nightmares: dreams that feel like glimpses into other lives, futures or realms. Unlike stress-related dreams, which are soaked in emotion, these dreams often feel matter-of-fact. You may dream of a departed loved one, a car crash or a strange detail and wake up with a sense of knowing, not fear.

Most dream experts don't think you can see the future in your dreams, but some believe that precognitive dreams are worth researching and should not be dismissed as coincidence. Visionary scientists such as Dr Julia Mossbridge have published encouraging results that appear to prove the idea of 'presentiment', which is when signals such as sweating and increased heart rate allow your body to sense what is going to take place before it actually happens.* So, if it is possible to sense the future when you are awake, might it also be possible to sense the future in your sleep?

Who knows. But if you consider that dreams challenge our perceptions about time because they take place outside measurable time – and science knows less about time and

* Julia Mossbridge et al., 'Predictive Physiological Anticipation Preceding Seemingly Unpredictable Stimuli: A Meta-Analysis', *Frontiers in Psychology*, 3 (2012), doi: 10.3389/fpsyg.2012.00390.

how it operates than it does about dreams – the possibility of glimpsing a potential future, sensing what cannot be sensed with our physical senses in our dreams, isn't as outlandish as it might seem. According to historians such as George Behe and Terry Keefe, there are well-known reports of dreams foretelling the sinking of the *Titanic*, and perhaps the most famous precognitive dream in history is that of US president Lincoln, who dreamed he saw his own dead body two weeks before he died. More recently, several people reported nightmarish dreams of chaos and destruction so realistic they woke up convinced a disaster was going to happen in the days before 9/11.

Signs of a psychic or precognitive dream include feeling emotionally flat but viscerally real. The dream may also be unusually detailed or timestamped – it may even have a beginning, middle and end, unlike symbolic dreams, which are like shapeshifting fragments. There will also be a sense of certainty or 'knowing' on waking.

As already discussed, though, the only way to know for sure whether a dream is truly precognitive or offering you a glimpse of the future is in hindsight. That is why it is vital to always date and timestamp your entries in your dream journal. You need to gather data and proof that your dreams are foreshadowing future events, bearing in mind that (in my humble opinion) every dream has precognitive elements in that they showcase your current mindset and the potential future it is attracting. The beauty of this is that if you don't like how your dream makes you feel on waking, this is your chance to attract a different future by changing your mindset.

Dreaming of a loved one's death shortly before it happens or having intense dreams during global disasters is well documented. As are shared dreams – where two people recall being in the same dream together, even miles apart. If you experience these kinds of psychic dreams, do not panic. Do not assume responsibility for the outcome. But do pay attention. Keep a dream diary. Mark the date. Document the details.

Over time, you may begin to recognize the texture of these dreams and how they differ from psychological or symbolic content. And that awareness can become a powerful inner compass. As a rule of thumb, to help you determine if a nightmare is symbolic, or literal, or potentially psychic, on waking first work through the seven-step dream-interpretation guide outlined in this book (see page 66) to see if it is a symbolic dream. If after that analysis you still feel uncertain, ask yourself the following questions:

- Was the dream emotional or did you feel removed from it? Remember, highly emotional dreams are often symbolic. Flat, eerie or precise dreams may be literal.
- Was the fear personal or more detached? If you felt deep fear but can't link it to an event, it's likely symbolic. If the

dream ignites a sense of knowing even though you can't explain why, it may be a warning.

- Was the dream rich in true-to-life details, such as people and places you recognize, and were characters' behaviours and reactions in the dream appropriate or realistic? If it was and they were, the chances are the dream was a psychic one.
- Was there a call to action? Some warning dreams feel instructional. You may wake up just knowing you must avoid a place, check on someone or take action. Trust that knowing.
- Did the dream repeat? Repeating dreams often point to inner change, not outer events. But if the content sharpens or becomes more specific and urgent in tone, take note.

Then ask your dreaming mind to send you another dream the following night to clarify. As you fall asleep you can revisit that initial dream and ask if it is a literal warning or not. Notice what dreams you recall in response the following morning.

The goal here is to cultivate discernment. Become your own dream detective. As already noted, most dreams are metaphor and not literal warnings and should be approached as such. This doesn't make them any less significant, as your dreaming mind is using imagery to draw your attention to something important in your life, such as a mindset that isn't working for you, a relationship that is toxic or a situation that is heading in the wrong direction for you. But when dreams are not literal, your inner wisdom often lets you know on waking or in the coming days when some element of your dream plays out. Trust it because it trusts you.

A Dream Remembered

According to the Sleep Foundation, between 18 and 38 per cent of people have experienced a precognitive dream;* while other research suggests the phenomenon is far more common than we think and may have been experienced by up to 97 per cent of us.†

As mentioned earlier, déjà rêvé, or 'already dreamed', is when you are going about your day and suddenly something – a person, a colour, an emotion, a symbol or anything else – brings your dream right back into your mind. You get a sense you have been here before, not as in déjà vu but in your dreams.

I have lost count of the number of times people have written to me over the years about elements of their dreams that have played out, usually within a few days but sometimes weeks, months or even years later. It is far more common than you think and this is why, as I previously noted, I have concluded

---

* Jay Vera Summer, 'What Are Precognitive (Premonition) Dreams?', *Sleep Doctor*, 14 July 2025 <https://www.sleepfoundation.org/dreams/precognitive-dreams> [accessed 20 November 2025].

† Julia Childs Heyl, 'When Dreams Merge with Your Waking Life – What to Know About Deja Reve', *Very Well Mind*, 20 November 2025 <https://www.verywellmind.com/deja-reve-8704831> [accessed 20 November 2025].

that every dream has precognitive elements: they mirror your mindset and the potential future that mindset is attracting. No wonder déjà rêvé is the norm, rather than the exception, if you don't change your mindset following a disturbing dream.

A powerful way to let your dreaming mind know that you believe in its psychic potential is to consciously create déjà rêvé. During the day, seek out an element of your dream – a colour, an object – that is safe and make contact with it. For example, if you dreamed of a seashore, go visit one in person or look at pictures of beaches online. Connecting with your dream in this proactive way can feel deeply sacred and lets your dreaming mind know you are not afraid of its ability to transcend space and time. You are consciously bringing your unconscious and conscious worlds together in a moment of sacred reflection.

Dream Telepathy

Telepathy is a word used to describe purported information obtained by one individual from another, supposedly through mind-to-mind contact. And unsurprisingly, there is a wealth of anecdotal evidence to suggest that this can and does happen in the dream state.

Dreams dissolve the barriers of time, space and ego, offering us a more fluid and receptive state of consciousness. Our waking mind relaxes its grip, allowing intuitive and psychic impressions to rise to the surface. While awake, we may filter or dismiss subtle mental impressions, but when we dream, we are wide open, unguarded receivers of the invisible signals that flow between minds. This is why dream telepathy is not only possible but may also be our most natural state of communication.

To explore this for yourself, try this simple exercise:

- Before sleeping, think of someone you feel closely connected to. Hold their image gently in your mind and silently 'send' them a loving, clear message or question.
- Upon waking, write down any dreams you recall, no matter how fragmented.
- Later, ask the person if they experienced anything unusual in their own dreams or feelings that night. With consistency and openness, you may notice meaningful overlaps, glimpses of true dream telepathy.

And if someone else appears in your dreams out of the blue, there is no harm done if you feel comfortable doing so telling them you dreamed of them. Most people find that very flattering to hear that they have made a cameo in your dreams, and you never know, you may have picked up on something and perhaps they were also dreaming about you.

Near-Death Visions

Of course, there can be no dream as extreme or 'out there' as a near-death experience (NDE) dream, when someone has clinically died, their brain and heart have stopped working and yet they return with vivid memories of what they believe to be visions of the afterlife. These experiences defy scientific explanation and yet are remarkably consistent across cultures, religions and ages. A hallmark of these experiences is not only the clarity and detail with which they are remembered but also their lasting emotional and spiritual impact. People emerge from them changed, more compassionate, more curious and often with a renewed sense of purpose.

Daniel and Charlotte: near-death experiences

Most NDEs are peaceful and filled with love and light. Take for example the case of Daniel, a firefighter who reached out to me to tell me about the miraculous vision he experienced after suffering cardiac arrest during a rescue mission. While doctors worked to revive him, Daniel recalls being enveloped in a warm, radiant light and meeting deceased relatives and angels who offered messages of comfort and encouragement. When he awoke, he no longer feared death and felt a deep desire to serve others on a more soulful level.

But not all experiences are blissful. Charlotte, a young woman who overdosed in her teens and spent days in a medically induced coma, described to me a petrifying descent into a dark, oppressive realm where she was plagued by feelings of isolation and dread. There were no demons, just an overwhelming sense of being lost and forgotten. Yet even this hellish vision proved transformative. Charlotte turned her life around completely, seeking therapy, reconnecting with her family and dedicating herself to healing herself and others, so that when her time to pass came she would do so without regrets.

Both the heavenly and the harrowing types of NDEs seem to act as a mirror, reflecting back what lies unprocessed or undiscovered within the psyche. Do they prove the existence of heaven or hell? No one can say for certain. Scientific proof of an afterlife still eludes us. But the power of these near-death stories is undeniable. They suggest that when the body and brain are suspended in limbo, consciousness may continue venturing into realms outside of time, where the journey of growth, healing and unconditional love continues, even beyond the final breath.

Are these extraordinary NDEs dreams or glimpses of something more? Science doesn't have a definitive answer. Some researchers argue that NDEs are vivid hallucinations caused by a lack of oxygen or creative spikes of brain activity in the final moments of life. But hallucinations typically cause disorientation and*

* Jessica M Lust et al., 'Activation of Mirror Neuron Regions Is Altered in Developmental Coordination Disorder (DCD) – Neurophysiological Evidence Using an Action Observation Paradigm', *Frontiers in Human Neuroscience*, 13 (2019), doi: 10.3389/fnhum.2019.00232.

depression, whereas NDEs have the opposite effect. Meanwhile other research, such as science of consciousness (noetic) studies, suggest that the richness, structure and lasting impact of NDEs point to something beyond biology. Unlike typical dreams, NDEs – and other psychic dreams – are often remembered with remarkable clarity years later and experiencers rarely view them as 'just dreams'. The truth may lie somewhere in between; perhaps these experiences represent a dreamlike threshold where consciousness begins to separate and move on from the body.*

This brings us to out-of-body experiences (OBEs), another phenomenon reported during trauma, sleep, NDEs or meditation. In OBEs, people describe floating outside their physical form, sometimes observing their own bodies from above. Some even report travelling to distant places or dimensions. Closely related is the idea of astral travel, where the dreamer intentionally leaves their body to explore other realms. Are these just vivid, lucid dreams or flights of imagination? Or are they subtle journeys of the soul? Science often categorizes them as altered states of consciousness, possibly rooted in neurological shifts during sleep or near-death. But for those who experience them, they can feel more real than waking life and like NDEs, they often change lives forever.

---

* Jeffrey Long and Marjorie Woollacott, 'Long-term Transformational Effects of Near-Death Experiences', *Explore*, 20(5) (2024), doi: 10.1016/j.explore.2024.103030.

If it Bleeds, it Leads

But you don't need to 'die' to discover the life-changing power of a vision in a dream. Nightmares, whether psychic or not, also can change your life for the better. You just need to not do everything you can to distract yourself and brush them aside on waking. Fortunately, this shouldn't be too difficult to do as the more alarming the dream the more likely you are to remember it and want to get to the bottom of it.

There's an old saying in journalism: 'If it bleeds, it leads.' It's meant cynically – bad news grabs attention, sells papers and dominates headlines. But as this book has illustrated, the phrase applies to our dreams too. When we wake from sleep, it's often the most disturbing, the most vivid, the most emotionally charged dream fragments that rise to the surface first.

You probably know the feeling. A happy dream of dancing in a meadow evaporates the moment your alarm goes off, but the image of being chased, betrayed or buried alive clings to your chest like smoke. You may remember just one dream out of the dozens you had that night and it's the one that made your heart pound. This isn't a flaw in your brain. It's a feature. It's ancient.

From an evolutionary perspective, being primed to remember threatening scenarios may once have kept us alive. If your dreaming brain simulated a tiger in the tall grass or a dangerous fall from a cliff, you were more likely to survive by being hyper-vigilant the next day.

This negativity bias is hardwired. It helped our ancestors stay alert. But in the modern world, where the threat isn't a predator but an email or an identity crisis, that same mechanism leaves us waking in anxiety, confusion or fear. And yet we don't have to stay there. We can interrupt that pattern the moment we open our eyes.

We can train ourselves to remember more than just the 'bleeding' imagery. We can choose to decode the symbolic nightmare not as a warning of doom but as a guidepost for healing. We can actively mine even the most upsetting dream for truth, wisdom and transformation. In doing so, we take back the morning. We take back our mood. And over time, we take back our own power because recalling your dreams encourages you to raise your waking vibration to attract what we want – not what we don't want – into our lives.

And yet it is still natural to wonder: Why are so many of my dreams upsetting? Why can't I just dream of love and magic and beautiful things? The answer, while not always comforting, is profoundly empowering: your dreams reflect the mindset you're outgrowing or what needs to be shed at a deep unconscious level, before you can make space from within for what is meant for you.

Nightmares and 'bad' dreams bring to the surface our deepest limiting beliefs, unconscious fears and wounds and repressed emotions and untended inner conflicts. They are mirrors to the darkest corners of our inner world not to shame us but to liberate us. A dream where you are voiceless may symbolize the part of you that has never been allowed to speak and which is in the process of dying. A dream of being lost may reflect your disorientation in waking life and the inner compass that is trying to be heard. A dream where your childhood home is crumbling may signal an outdated belief system cracking open.

These dreams show you the inner workings of your suffering, so you can face it, understand it and then let go of it with compassion and make space in your inner world for light. In this way, dreamwork becomes the ultimate inside-out healing technology and the original and best pre-manifestation tool.

Dreamwork as Manifestation

If you've ever heard the phrase, 'Where your attention goes, your energy flows', then you understand the core principle of manifestation: what you focus on is the energy you magnify and attract to you.

Dreams give us the blueprint of our current energetic focus. They show us, in symbolic language, what we are rehearsing emotionally and energetically beneath the surface. For example, a recurring nightmare of failure? You may be carrying an old identity rooted in unworthiness. A dream of a closed door? Perhaps there's a belief in limitation you haven't challenged. A dream of death? It could be a version of yourself dying, making room for the next.

When we decode our darkest dreams with feelings of unconditional love, we gain the opportunity to rewrite the story we unconsciously believe about ourselves and what is possible for us. Every time we bring awareness to a limiting unconscious belief revealed to us in a dream, we loosen its unconscious energetic grip on us in waking life. Dreamwork becomes not just a mirror but a magnet.

And the better we understand the terrain of our dreams, the more consciously we can understand ourselves and start to create inner shifts in response to what our dreams reveal to us. What you unconsciously believe is what your dreams reveal to you and what you may tend to attract in waking life. Your brain doesn't know the difference between experiencing something in the dream state and in waking life, so if you can dream it, it believes you can do it – and when you have that level of inside-out belief anything is possible. And on that high note it is high time now to lose your fear not just of dying and falling in your dreams but also of flying in them.

Flying Dreams

Although most of our dreams will have a dark tone, for the reasons explained above, you can shift that. In the past you may have occasionally woken up from something luminous, a dream of flying, dancing, kissing or laughing. You may have felt weightless, free or full of joy. These dreams are rare not because they are unnatural but because our culture tends to undervalue bliss. We are trained to worry, not to soar. From now on, whenever you do wake up with a beautiful dream in your chest, please, please pause for a moment to celebrate it. Write it down. Revisit it many times over during the day and the following day. Let the feeling of the dream spill into your waking actions.

These dreams are not frivolous. They are affirmations of your soul's natural state: joy, creativity, connection. They show you what's possible when fear is quiet. The more you honour them, the more often they will come. Because yes, the happier your dreams, the happier your life.

Looking Back at You

To paraphrase psychic Edgar Cayce, the future is always looking back at you in your dreams. Every dream you have reflects your current mindset and the future it is attracting. Every dream is an opportunity to course correct by changing your current mindset if need be. Every dream is an invitation to attract a beautiful future or good things.

So, the future of your dreams, both the 'bad' and the good ones, is to take the precious wisdom you have learned here and apply it in your waking life so you can start feeling and living the benefits.

But don't stop there – share what you have learned here with your loved ones and anyone willing to listen. I dream of a future where dreamwork is taught in schools so that from an early age children will have a connection to the transformative and healing power of their inner world – and this connection to their soul will give them a sense of self-confidence, fulfilment and purpose unlike any other. I dream of a day when the medical profession prescribes dream therapy and when dreamwork is used as a healing tool in prisons and hospitals.

And I dream of a future when the whole world wakes up with night visions and gratitude for them on their mind. A world where dreamwork connects and does not divide us; and reminds us that we are all dreaming beings having a human experience. Because whoever you are and whatever your belief or recall, one thing is certain: you are going to need to sleep every single night – and whenever you fall asleep you are going to dream.

Healing Dream Practices

Here are a few more gentle guided daily practices to reinforce the idea that all of your dreams – the good, the bad and the ugly – are energetic portals to your own healing and manifestation.

The morning rewrite

As soon as you wake up, journal any dreams on your mind from an observational or third-person perspective. Ask yourself: 'What part of me or aspect of my waking life did this dream reflect? What was I believing about myself in this dream? Where did that belief originate and is it still true?'

This brings your subconscious programming into the light. Awareness is the first step in dismantling it. Then feel nothing but love for the dream and write a second version where the outcome is empowered. This practice helps rewire the brain and turns fear into conscious authorship. You're reminding your subconscious: 'I'm not powerless here. I can direct what is going on inside me and what it is attracting into my waking life.'

Nightly affirmation ritual

Each night before bed, place your hands over your stomach and say: 'Tonight, I dream with clarity. I meet all parts of myself with love. I welcome guidance and transformation.'

This sets the tone for gentle, healing dreams and reorients your nervous system towards trust. Then close your eyes and imagine or feel a chalice or cauldron glowing at the centre of your being. Into it, pour all fears, dreams, regrets and imagine them transmuting into light. Say: 'I release. I transform. I become.'

This nightly ritual teaches your subconscious that even pain can become power and can be transformed into purpose.

Daily dream-empowerment reflection

Begin and end each day by sitting quietly for a few moments. Take three deep, slow breaths, allowing yourself to settle into a calm and open space.

In essence, you are the creator of your dreams. Your dreaming mind is your own masterpiece and a reflection of you, mirroring your thoughts, feelings and choices. Every night, your mind weaves stories to showcase to you the state of your inner world – your hopes, fears and imagination. Remember what this book has repeatedly stressed: your dreams do not happen to you. They just reflect you without judgement for the purpose of helping you heal and grow.

If a dream or nightmare feels frightening, know that these experiences are not trying to harm you. Your dreaming mind is your best friend, always seeking to surprise and guide you. Sometimes dreams in their honesty turn the nightlight on inner challenges and blocks to help you grow, but they come from a place of love and learning.

In the rare moments when dreams seem psychic, know this too comes from a realm of love offering insight and connection beyond the everyday. Trust that your inner mind supports and protects you always.

Whenever you wake from a crazy dream, gently affirm: 'I am safe. I create my dreams with my thoughts and choices. I have the power to love the message of that dream and choose how I respond.' You can choose to see your dreams as opportunities to understand yourself better, not as threats.

Avoid getting stuck in any dream analysis that drags you down. Instead, embrace the universally unacknowledged truth that you are the author of your dreamworld, a world shaped by your mindset and decisions; and it is your choice, moving forward, to always interpret your dreams with a positive perspective.

Each day and every night, take your dreams seriously and as much as possible nurture kindness and love towards them and therefore yourself. With this newfound compassionate relationship with your dreaming mind, your fear will soften, replaced by fascination and confidence in your power to create a peaceful, inspiring dreamlife.

Nothing could be simpler: falling in love with your dreams is falling in love with your essence, your inner world, who you truly are. Dreamwork is a sacred act of self-care and self-respect.

All the Wonders That Can Be

This book has made it crystal clear that your dreams are a nightly unfolding of your personal, psychic and spiritual evolution. They reveal where you are stuck, where you are strong, where you are ready to bloom.

Extreme dreams are feedback. They show us the places that still ache for understanding, still long for freedom. When you begin to work with your dreams – all of them, from the terrifying to the transcendent – you begin to work with your intuition directly. And something shifts.

You become more self-aware, which leads to more self-love, which blossoms over time into deep self-belief. And from that sacred place? Your life – forgive the pun but dreams do love to pun and play with creative ways to showcase your mindset – becomes a waking dream.

Your dreaming self and your waking self are not separate. They are one. You are still you in a dream; just in a different state of consciousness. And from this awareness of yourself as a dreaming being you can take another giant leap forward from the inside out. Moving forward, you can interpret everything and everyone in your waking life in the same way you would interpret and work with a nocturnal dream. You can look beneath the surface of everyone for deeper levels of meaning. You can understand when you are projecting your own mindset. You can take back your own power with your evolving awareness that your perception creates your reality in every moment. You can connect to the intelligence of your emotions and all your dreams. You can constantly open your mind and ask questions of yourself and the true meaning of your life.

And the beauty of living in this dream-inspired way is that you will not only be going to places you have never been before but you will also be going with the instinct of your brain, which is to forever seek meaning and a sense of connection in everyone and in everything. There is another way to describe this. It is bliss.

7

101 NIGHTMARE SYMBOLS AND THEIR SECRET MEANINGS

Every nightmare, no matter how unsettling, carries a secret meaning that is longing to be exposed. This chapter offers an alphabetical guide to 101 of the most commonly reported nightmare symbols, drawn from dream research across the world, along with interpretations to help you see their light.

You may wonder why 101. It's a deliberate choice, inspired by Orwell's Room 101 from his classic novel *1984* – the place where deepest fears are faced. Think of this chapter as your own symbolic Room 101. Not to terrify but to illuminate. Not to punish but to empower. These 101 symbols reflect the nightmares most of us are likely to encounter at some point in our lives, and each one is a unique stepping stone to greater awareness.

Of course, this book can't include every nightmare you might experience. Nowhere can – apart from the mystical Akashic Records, perhaps, which are believed to capture the dreams of everyone and everything. The hallmark of a nightmare is simply that it is personally frightening – but bear in mind one person's nightmare symbol may not be another's. What scares someone in waking life and in their dreams may not scare someone else. If your dream doesn't match a listed word exactly, simply look for broader themes to kickstart your symbolic interpretation. For example, an ogre might fall under 'monsters', a hurricane under 'natural disasters'. Trust your instincts to guide your search.

Nightmares aren't random. They're emotional messengers on a mission to reveal what's hidden in the shadows of your psyche. They confront us not to scare us but to awaken us. They highlight what we've ignored, repressed or feared to face. Interpreting them isn't about finding one fixed answer; it's about uncovering layers of deeper meaning to help you ask better questions and discover more about your own potential for personal growth. The right interpretation is the one that helps you grow, offers clarity or shifts your perspective or surprises you. If an explanation feels heavy or hopeless, it may not be the right one for you.

Nightmares are sacred invitations to better understand yourself and from that inner exploration to evolve into a higher version of yourself. Real change can begin only when you stop running from what scares you and start listening to what it's trying to tell you. This simple inner shift – from alarm to curiosity, from avoidance to courage – can turn even your darkest dreams into powerful allies for your personal and spiritual growth. With that in mind, let's open the door to our Room 101 and the nightfrights cowering inside it.

Content Warning:

This book explores 101 symbols drawn from nightmares and the darker corners of the human psyche. Some entries include themes that may be deeply distressing, including sexual violence, abuse, fear and loss of control. Reader discretion is strongly advised. Please take care while engaging with this material, and feel free to pause or skip sections if needed to protect your wellbeing.

101 Extreme-Dreaming Scenarios

1. Abuse

Nightmares of abuse highlight areas in your life where power has been lost, misused or violated, either by others or by your own self-talk. The abuser may symbolize a real person or your inner critic. These dreams aren't here to retraumatize but to help you reclaim your own power.

Ask yourself: 'Where in my life do I feel voiceless or unsafe? How do I betray myself through silence or self-blame?'

Self-help: Begin with small acts of self-empowerment. Set clear boundaries. Stop giving away your power to others or diminishing yourself. Challenge any voice that tears you down.

2. Alien

The alien may represent parts of yourself you've disowned – desires, fears or changes you can't yet recognize. This is less about outer space and more about inner disconnection.

Ask yourself: 'What part of me feels strange or unacceptable? Where am I struggling to belong?'

Self-help: Welcome the unfamiliar. Explore what you fear or reject through writing, art or talking with someone safe. Integration – understanding that you are the source of your own power – takes time, but it starts with curiosity. Your dream isn't about being invaded; it's about becoming whole.

3. Ambush

Nightmares of ambush point to hidden stress or emotional overwhelm catching you off guard. Whether it's conflict, anxiety or pressure, something has crept up uninvited. Sometimes, the ambusher is your own racing thoughts.

Ask yourself: 'What am I avoiding that is urgent? Where do I feel blindsided or unprotected?'

Self-help: Ground yourself. Build routines that create a sense of safety. Address what you've postponed, one step at a time. Ambush dreams don't predict disaster; they call for presence, preparation and calm in the storm.

4. Anger

Anger themes in your nightmares reveal buried frustrations – rage you've swallowed or avoided out of guilt or fear. You may fear losing control, but your dream says something needs to be expressed.

Ask yourself: 'Where am I denying or downplaying my feelings? What needs to be said or changed?'

Self-help: Make space for emotion without shame. Use movement, journalling or honest dialogue to release it constructively. Anger is a messenger, not a monster. Let it speak so it doesn't have to scream in your nightmares.

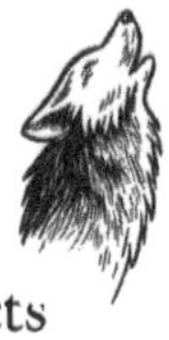

5. Animals (wild/aggressive)

Being chased or attacked by wild animals in dreams reflects human emotions that feel overwhelming – instincts, fears or desires that can't be tamed by logic. They aren't enemies; they're instinctive parts of you demanding to be felt.

Ask yourself: 'What powerful impulse have I been trying to suppress? Do I recognize these basic instincts in myself?'

Self-help: Get back in touch with your body and with nature. Dance, scream, run, create. These dreams aren't threats; they're wakeup calls to rewild your inner life and reconnect with feelings you've caged for too long.

6. Apocalypse

Apocalyptic nightmares mirror emotional collapse or radical life changes on the horizon that may soon be beyond your control. Something in your waking life – beliefs, identity or relationships – may be falling apart. It feels final, but it's also a threshold.

Ask yourself: 'What's ending that I haven't acknowledged? What am I afraid to say goodbye to?'

Self-help: Focus on essentials. Let go of the non-urgent, find comfort in simplicity. Change is disruptive, but it also clears space for better things. This dream isn't just about destruction of what is familiar – it's about survival and rebirth. Begin again, one grounded step at a time.

7. Attack/being attacked

Nightmares of attacks/being attacked physically or verbally reveal where you feel unsafe – emotionally, physically or psychologically. The attacker may represent external threats or your own inner judge. You're being shown where protection is needed.

Ask yourself: 'Who or what is threatening my inner peace? How well do I express what angers me?'

Self-help: Rebuild your inner fortress. Practise saying no. Learn to pause before reacting. This dream calls for stronger boundaries and self-trust. You have the right to defend your energy and your space.

8. Bites

Bite nightmares hint at emotional injuries – small, sharp, often unexpected. You may be tolerating something toxic or ignoring subtle violations of trust. The bite says that something in your life is gradually eating away at you. A dog biting in a dream suggests that someone or something once loving and loyal no longer is.

Ask yourself: 'What pain have I been minimizing? Who or what disarms me in quiet, repeated ways?'

Self-help: Be honest about what hurts, even if it seems small. Speak up, walk away or set limits. Pay more attention to the actions rather than the words of others.

9. Blood

Nightmares featuring blood signal emotional exhaustion or deep wounds. Whether from heartbreak, burnout or sacrifice, your life force is leaking.

Ask yourself: 'What's draining my energy or passion? Where am I giving too much?'

Self-help: Rest is not indulgence – it's survival. Reclaim your energy through sleep, nourishment and emotional boundaries. Dreams about blood on your hands or everywhere aren't just gruesome and unsettling; they're vital warnings to care for your essence now before you lose too much strength.

10. Broken bones

Dreams of broken bones reflect inner collapse or feeling unsupported, unstable or emotionally fractured. Something fundamental feels damaged, whether it's your confidence, relationships or sense of identity.

Ask yourself: 'What part of me is struggling to hold it together? Where do I need support?'

Self-help: Let yourself break and then rebuild. Ask for support, reduce your load and give time to what hurts. Healing is messy, but broken bones fuse stronger at the break. Your dream says you must pause. Regroup. You're not weak – you're wounded and need time to repair.

Broken-bones nightmare – Luis

Luis dreamed repeatedly of his bones shattering under the strain of carrying heavy loads. The physical pain lingered even after waking. In reality, he was emotionally overwhelmed: recovering from divorce, balancing single parenting and facing work burnout.

The dream's symbolism became clear: the breaking bones reflected his exhaustion and emotional fragility. Through therapy, Luis recognized how little support he was giving himself. He set clearer work boundaries, joined a parenting group and allowed himself rest.

As he rebuilt emotional strength and learned to ask for help, the nightmares subsided. His dream was a wakeup call: he didn't need to carry everything alone.

11. Buried alive

Being buried alive in a nightmare expresses extreme overwhelm – expectations, grief or shame pressing down until you can barely breathe. Yet even in the dark, something in you resists. That's your will to live freely.

Ask yourself: 'What is suffocating my true self? Whose approval am I chasing at my own expense?'

Self-help: Begin un-burying yourself. Say 'no more', breathe deeply, speak honestly. Let go of roles that feel like coffins. You don't have to live for others. Your dream is a rebellion against being silenced. Make sure you honour it by coming back to life.

12. Cannibalism

Cannibalism in nightmares reflects being consumed by others' needs, guilt or self-sacrifice and lines being crossed. Sometimes, it's about internal destruction, where one part of you devours another in shame or inner conflict.

Ask yourself: 'Who is draining me emotionally or energetically? How am I turning against myself?'

Self-help: Start nourishing your needs instead of feeding everyone else's. Reclaim your time, space and voice. Choose restoration over depletion. Stop giving yourself away piece by piece and practise self-care before you disappear under the weight of expectation or guilt.

13. Car crashes

Crash and accident themes in dreams signal life feeling out of control emotionally, mentally or even physically – and that if the direction your life is heading in doesn't shift there could be a sudden shock. You might be speeding towards burnout, ignoring red lights or letting someone else drive you into the ground.

Ask yourself: 'Where have I lost control in my life? Am I making decisions aligned with who I really am?'

Self-help: Slow down. Reflect before reacting. Realign with your values and path. The dream isn't a premonition – it's a red flag. Whether you're the driver or passenger matters: are you in charge of the direction of your life or handing over the wheel?

14. Caught in the act

Dreams of being caught red-handed – lying, stealing, hiding – point to shame, guilt or fear of being truly seen. They often surface when you're living out of alignment with your truth or feeling like an imposter.

Ask yourself: 'What am I hiding from myself and others? Where am I not being honest with myself?'

Self-help: Tell yourself the truth first. Then share it safely with compassion, not judgement. These dreams are not punishments; they're requests for authenticity. Real peace comes not from hiding but from being seen and accepted even by yourself.

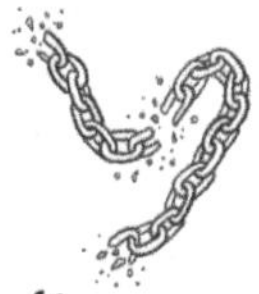

15. Chains

Nightmares of chains, ropes or handcuffs symbolize emotional captivity and resulting limiting beliefs, toxic dynamics or fears that restrict your freedom. You may feel stuck, helpless or weighed down.

Ask yourself: 'What or who is keeping me bound? Am I trapping myself with guilt, fear or old roles?'

Self-help: Awareness loosens the grip. Name what's holding you back, then take one bold step towards freedom. Say no, set a boundary or speak an unspoken truth. Liberation begins not with escape but with reclaiming your right to live unchained.

16. Chased

Being chased in nightmares means you're running from something that makes you feel vulnerable – an emotion, memory, truth or even your own potential. The more you run, the more powerful it feels.

Ask yourself: 'What feels too overwhelming to face? What part of me is trying to get my attention?'

Self-help: Pause and turn around, even just mentally. Imagine what would happen if you stopped running. Often, the threat reveals a message or unmet need. These dreams call for courage, not escape. You don't need to fight – you just need to listen and respond with compassion.

Chased nightmare – Aisha

Aisha had recurring nightmares of being chased through dark alleys by a faceless figure. Each time, she awoke panicked. In real life, she was avoiding the emotional fallout from a breakup and overwhelming work stress.

With support, Aisha explored the dream's meaning and saw the shadow as her own suppressed anxiety. Journalling and mindfulness helped her identify the emotions she had been running from – sadness, fear and guilt. She gradually opened up difficult conversations with her ex and her boss.

As she faced these unresolved issues, the nightmares eased. Aisha's dream revealed what she'd been avoiding emotionally, and by turning towards her fear, she began to reclaim a sense of control and peace.

17. Cheating

Nightmares of yourself cheating or betraying others highlight potential self-betrayal and lack of self-respect. These dreams may mirror parts of your waking life where you're compromising your values, silencing your truth or living inauthentically to gain approval or avoid conflict.

Ask yourself: 'Where do I feel unsafe, unloved or unseen? What promises have I made to myself that I continue to break, whether through fear, people-pleasing or self-doubt?'

Self-help: Stop settling for scraps and seek the honesty and care you deserve. Begin by honouring your inner voice in small ways each day – setting clear boundaries, speaking your truth and making choices that reflect self-loyalty over external validation.

18. Child in danger

A baby, child or young animal in extreme danger or being neglected in nightmares represents vulnerable parts of you, your inner child, creative spark or sense of joy and innocence that feel threatened or neglected.

Ask yourself: 'What vulnerable part of me needs protection or healing? What commitments are not working out?'

Self-help: Make space for softness. Rest, play, laugh, cry. Your dream is a reminder to nurture yourself with extreme care, as you would a beloved child. That part of you isn't weak; it's bursting with creativity and it needs nurturing to thrive again.

19. Clowns

Clown nightmares often represent discomfort with artificial personas, either your own or someone else's. They can also reflect fear of being seen as foolish or fake.

Ask yourself: 'Where am I performing or joking around instead of being real? Who in my life once brought joy but now feels inauthentic?'

Self-help: Be brave enough to take off the mask. Choose truth over perfection, depth over performance. These dreams encourage realness and no more pretending everything's fine when it's not. You don't need to play a part. Just be who you are, mess and all. You are enough.

20. Collapse (houses, buildings, structures)

Dreams of collapsing structures reveal internal instability. Something that once held you up – an identity, belief or relationship – no longer feels solid and reliable. The foundation is crumbling.

Ask yourself: 'What part of my life no longer supports me? What am I afraid to let fall apart?'

Self-help: Let the collapse happen. It's not failure – it's release, so that something new can be built in its place. Clear the rubble, grieve the loss and start again with stronger, truer foundations. Your dream is clearing space. Trust that something greater is waiting to be built.

21. Confined spaces

Nightmares of tight or suffocating spaces reflect extreme emotional or situational pressure in your waking life. You may feel trapped by expectations, routines or internalized fear.

Ask yourself: 'Where am I shrinking to stay safe? What needs more space to grow in my life?'

Self-help: Create more room emotionally, physically, creatively. Say no. Take a break. Speak up. Your dream shows you're too confined to thrive right now. Start stretching into the space you deserve. Breathe slowly and deeply through your nose rather than your mouth. Even changing the way that you breathe can begin the transformation.

22. Darkness

Being lost in darkness or fog symbolizes uncertainty, fear or emotional blindness. These nightmares often arise when you're unsure of what's next or resisting inner truths that can help you see yourself more clearly.

Ask yourself: 'What am I avoiding or refusing to see? What truth lies just beyond my fear?'

Self-help: Instead of fearing the unknown, explore it gently. Use dreams, journalling or meditation to feel your way forward. The dark isn't always danger – it's a doorway. Step through slowly, with inquisitiveness. Trust that your inner light will guide you.

23. Death

Death-dream themes – funerals, graves, coffins, tombstones – (see Chapter Five) represent not an ending but a transformation. Something old – an identity, relationship, habit – is being released so that something new can grow.

Ask yourself: 'What needs to end for me to move forward? What have I outgrown but not let go of yet?'

Self-help: Let yourself grieve. Letting go can be sublime – just look at the beauty of autumn leaves. Say goodbye through ritual, journalling or silence. These dreams say you should trust the cycle of darkness before the dawn. What feels like death may just be rebirth. Let go to grow.

24. Demons/devils

Demonic nightmare themes reflect intense internal battles with guilt, shame, anger, lust, envy or other negative urges you've buried. These figures represent exiled parts of you crying out to be seen and understood. It is time to confront what terrifies you.

Ask yourself: 'What feeling or part of myself have I judged as evil? What do I fear about facing it?'

Self-help: Shadow work is key here. Approach your demons with compassion, not fear. Talk with a therapist, if need be, or journal with absolute honesty. The goal isn't to destroy your dark parts; it's to integrate them. Only through understanding can your inner demons become guides instead of tormentors.

25. Disasters

Dreams featuring natural disasters can symbolize upheavals you've been trying to contain. Rather than just work or relationship stress, these dreams may reflect a larger internal shift or transformation trying to break through. Something long held may be ready to collapse so something more authentic can emerge.

Ask yourself: 'What internal structures or beliefs are being challenged or eroded? Where am I trying to maintain control while something greater is demanding change?'

Self-help: Rather than resisting, try to listen to what the chaos is revealing. Breathe deeply. Connect with your body through movement or stillness. Express what's surfacing through words, art or action. These dreams may not just warn but initiate. Let them guide you to what's waiting beneath the surface.

26. Drowning

Drowning dreams show you're emotionally overwhelmed or silently struggling beneath the surface. You may feel pulled under by stress, grief or responsibility.

Ask yourself: 'What emotion is too heavy to carry alone? Where am I pretending I'm fine when I'm not?'

Self-help: Stop battling the current. Give yourself time to breathe. Ask for support. Let yourself feel what you've been holding back. These dreams are cries for relief. They reveal what needs your attention and compassion before it pulls you in too deep.

Drowning nightmare – Priya

Priya had horrifying dreams of drowning in deep water, unable to breathe. Upon waking, she felt panic and fatigue.

In waking life, she was juggling a high-pressure job, caregiving for her terminally ill mother and managing her own growing anxiety.

Through therapy, Priya understood the water symbolized emotional overwhelm. She asked herself, 'What am I holding in? Who can help me?'

She began setting boundaries, seeking support and practising mindfulness. Slowly, she stopped suppressing her feelings and learned to release them in healthy ways. The nightmares faded, replaced by moments of calm. Her dreams reminded her that she couldn't carry everything alone and didn't have to.

27. Earthquake

Dreams of earthquakes shake loose what's been hidden or buried but that needs to surface for your personal growth. A crumbling ground mirrors inner instability or a life structure collapsing under pressure.

Ask yourself: 'What belief, role or relationship no longer feels solid? What am I struggling to keep together?'

Self-help: Let it break. Not all damage is destruction, some clears space for growth. You're not losing ground; you're uncovering truth. Anchor yourself in the present while you rebuild stronger. This isn't the end of safety – it's the start of something real.

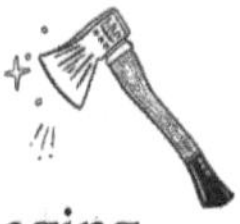

28. Execution

Execution dreams often signal forced endings or damaging levels of self-criticism. You may feel silenced, trapped or condemned – either by others or by your own inner critic.

Ask yourself: 'What truth am I killing off to please others? Why do I feel I always need to be perfect?'

Self-help: Release the role or belief that keeps you locked up. Let go of the pressure to be perfect. Forgive yourself for being a perfectly imperfect human. These dreams mark a turning point – this is not your death but the death of what's been stopping you growing.

29. Failure (test, project, work)

Failing in dreams rarely means failure in waking life. It reflects self-doubt, performance anxiety or fear of not being enough. It could also point to a responsibility that needs more preparation.

Ask yourself: 'What part of me is afraid I'll never measure up? Do I believe in myself or not?'

Self-help: Try. Fall. Learn. Get up again. These dreams remind you that growth is messy. You're not here to impress everyone; you're here to evolve. Let go of the need to prove yourself. Progress isn't perfection – it's persistence and learning and growing from your mistakes along the way. The only person you need to impress is the person you are going to be tomorrow.

30. Falling

Falling in dreams is the mind's way of expressing panic, lack of control, feeling unsupported or sudden instability. You may be in emotional free fall or feel you are losing your balance.

Ask yourself: 'Where do I feel unsupported or out of my depth? What in my life is heading for a fall?'

Self-help: Instead of bracing for certain impact, pause. Breathe. Focus on grounding and being mindful in the present. Find ways to support and trust yourself more. These dreams aren't about an inevitable crash – they're a signal that it's time to go with the flow, to float rather than fall to solid ground.

31. Fire

Fire and burning nightmares can signal inner change, not just destruction. Fire may represent destructive rage or intense desire as well as purification – a release of what no longer serves you. A wildfire in a dream might point to something internal that's outgrown its form and needs to be transformed.

Ask yourself: 'What is burning inside me? What needs to be released so something new can begin?'

Self-help: Don't suppress or deny what is burning inside you – channel it. Speak, move, create. Fire can destroy, but it can also renew. Let it strip away what's false so what's real can rise. Let the flames clear the way ahead, not consume it.

32. Flood

Dreams of floods are not just about water but about what's been held back. A flood in your dream can symbolize unspoken truths, repressed emotions or stress that's become too much to contain. You may be feeling stressed or emotionally overwhelmed, like you're just barely keeping your head above water.

Ask yourself: 'What feelings have I been suppressing? Where in my life am I nearing an emotional breaking point?'

Self-help: Let it out – cry, write, speak, scream if you must. These dreams aren't warnings of doom; they're *emotional release valves*. They show you what needs to move, to shift, to be felt. Flood dreams aren't something to fear. They're a signal: it's time to stop bottling things up. Let the emotional tide rise, not to drown you but to cleanse and free you.

33. Flying

In your dreams, fear of flying or losing control when you are flying without wings speaks to ambition outrunning stability. You may be chasing goals without a foundation or fearing failure at high altitude.

Ask yourself: 'What am I striving for without support? Where am I ignoring warning signs in pursuit of success?'

Self-help: Regroup. Slow down. Strengthen your base before you take off again. These dreams remind you that it's not just about rising above to see the bigger picture but about staying aligned with what grounds you. Learn to fly with balance, not just speed.

34. Forest

A dark or confusing forest in a dream signals emotional fog or a spiritual crossroads. You may be feeling lost and directionless in your waking life.

Ask yourself: 'Where am I unsure of my direction? What part of me feels hidden or ignored?'

Self-help: Don't rush the path. Slow down and listen. The forest holds wisdom. Let your intuition not fear lead the way. These dreams ask you to stop looking for the exit and start finding yourself inside the mystery. To focus on the journey and what it has to teach you about yourself rather than the destination.

35. Ghosts

Ghost dreams bring back what's unresolved – grief, regret or memories that still haunt. They signal the emotional past still echoing in the present.

Ask yourself: 'What or who have I not made peace with? What part of me feels stuck in yesterday?'

Self-help: Make space to process. Write letters, speak truths, allow goodbyes. Ghosts don't ask for fear; they ask to be witnessed. When acknowledged, they often fade. This is your big chance to lay something to rest, finally.

36. Guilt and punishment

Dreams of guilt or punishment reflect self-blame or unresolved shame. You may be stuck in a cycle of inner judgement, unable to forgive yourself.

Ask yourself: 'Am I punishing myself for making a mistake? Is this guilt helping me grow or just keeping me stuck?'

Self-help: Name the feeling. Accept your flaws. Take responsibility if needed, then let it go. These dreams urge you to stop carrying what's already been felt. Forgiveness is not forgetting – it's choosing not to suffer endlessly for the same mistake and to instead learn and grow wiser from it.

37. Halloween

Halloween-themed dreams point to disguise, performance or hiding your real self. You may be putting on emotional masks or not being true to yourself to feel accepted by others or safe.

Ask yourself: 'Who am I pretending to be? Can I laugh at my fears?'

Self-help: You don't have to unmask overnight. But begin noticing where you're not being honest with others or yourself. These dreams aren't spooky; they're invitations to drop the act and start showing up for real. They can also encourage you to lighten up, because if you can laugh at a fear it loses its power.

38. Haunted house

A haunted house in dreams reflects neglected parts of your inner world – memories, pain or emotions sealed behind closed doors.

Ask yourself: 'What part of myself have I shut away? What memory still echoes through my mind and needs to be put to rest?'

Self-help: Explore gently. There's no need to open every door at once. Begin with curiosity, not fear. Therapy, journalling or rituals can help you reclaim what's been buried. When you make peace with the haunted rooms, they become places of healing.

Haunted-house nightmare – Noah

Noah often dreamed of wandering through a crumbling, shadowy house that filled him with dread. In waking life, he was carrying unresolved childhood trauma and emotional neglect that he'd long buried.

The dream's haunted house mirrored his inner emotional landscape – broken, full of unspoken grief. With therapy, Noah faced these memories, exploring the rooms of his own past with care.

As he processed his pain and practised self-compassion, the dreams became less intense. The nightmare invited him to revisit what he had feared and avoided, ultimately helping him rebuild a sense of emotional safety within himself.

39. Hunted

Being hunted in dreams reveals pressure, fear or stress chasing you down in your waking life. If you're the hunter, you may be chasing something for fear of missing out rather than because you truly want it.

Ask yourself: 'Am I running from responsibility, fear or a part of myself? What am I pursuing and why?'

Self-help: Stop the chase. Face what's following you or question what you're chasing. The dream doesn't ask you to escape or capture – only to wake up and choose your path with intention, not panic.

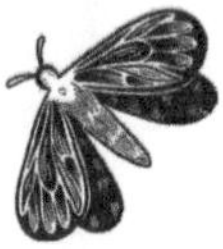

40. Insects

Insects in dreams – especially in swarms – symbolize mental clutter, anxiety or problems that are difficult to control but that you've minimized until they've multiplied.

Ask yourself: 'What little thing is becoming a big problem? What are you putting off addressing?'

Self-help: Take one issue at a time. Clean out the mental hive. Create to-do lists and stick to them. These dreams ask for small, steady action, not panic. Swat away daily stresses by creating space to breathe and practising time management. Even tiny steps can restore calm.

41. Intruder

An intruder in your home signals a deep violation – your emotional space, privacy or boundaries are being breached.

This nightmare often reflects anxiety about vulnerability, invasion or betrayal.

Ask yourself: 'Who or what is entering my life uninvited? Where am I ignoring red flags?'

Self-help: Reinforce your energetic and emotional boundaries. Say no without guilt. This dream isn't just fear – it's your psyche sounding the alarm. You are not powerless. Reclaim your space before something (or someone) claims it for you.

42. Jail or prison

Being imprisoned in a dream reveals that you may be headed in the wrong direction or that you are imprisoned by guilt, fear, outdated beliefs or roles you've outgrown.

Ask yourself: 'What self-imposed cage am I living in? What mindset is no longer serving me?'

Self-help: Challenge what keeps you confined. Let go of stories that say you can't change. This nightmare doesn't show you what you can't change; it shows you what you need to break free from. The door is open. Walk out.

Prison nightmare – Mike

Mike repeatedly dreamed of being locked in a dark, airless prison. He woke feeling trapped and hopeless. In real life, he was stuck in a creativity-stifling job and burdened by guilt over past decisions.

The dream prison symbolized emotional confinement. Mike asked: 'What regrets am I clinging to? What would freedom look like?'

Through therapy, he began forgiving himself, releasing shame and making small but empowering changes – taking on creative side projects and setting boundaries at work. As he reconnected with purpose, the dream prison dissolved. The nightmare marked the start of his emotional liberation.

43. Kidnapping

Kidnapping dreams are dreadful because they reflect stolen autonomy. You feel hijacked out of the blue by someone or something, either in your waking life or by your own past or fear itself.

Ask yourself: 'What part of me feels taken? Do I own my voice, time, truth or identity?'

Self-help: Take one small step towards reclaiming your power. Say what you mean. Choose what feels right. This nightmare isn't just about what's been taken; it's about waking up to the part of you that's always ready to fight for your freedom.

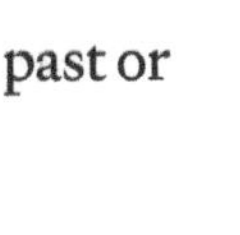

44. Knife or stabbing

Dreams of knives, scissors, cutting or stabbing are brutal emotional messages – betrayal, grief or rage that cuts deep and makes you bleed. Whether you're the attacker or the wounded, the pain is real.

Ask yourself: 'Where have I been pierced by sudden words or unexplained silence? What unresolved conflict is hurting me or cutting deep?'

Self-help: Don't ignore the bleeding. Speak the pain, name the wound. This dream points to what needs to be severed or healed. Pain doesn't vanish when buried; it festers. Honesty is the scalpel that frees you.

45. Lice or parasites

Parasites in nightmares reflect what's feeding on you: toxic people, shame, guilt or draining habits. Small things have become invasive and potentially toxic.

Ask yourself: 'What or who in my life is quietly devouring my energy? In what area of my life am I giving more than I am receiving?'

Self-help: Cleanse mentally, emotionally, physically. Remove what clings to you out of habit, not health. These dreams aren't gross for no reason, they demand action. Stop tolerating the itch. Purge whatever poisons you or drags you down. Peace begins with subtraction.

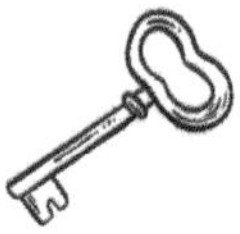

46. Losing something important

Nightmares of loss – your child, bag, voice, wallet, property, wealth or identity – echo the fear that something vital is slipping away in your waking life. It's not just about the object; it's about what it represents.

Ask yourself: 'What loss am I dreading? Where do I feel at risk?'

Self-help: Take stock of what really matters. These dreams don't predict loss – they urge you to focus on what truly matters and not getting your self-worth from other people and things. Reconnect with what grounds you. Sometimes, losing something in a dream means you're being asked to find yourself again.

47. Lost

Being lost in a nightmare reflects confusion or emotional crisis. You may feel directionless, especially when old paths no longer seem to lead anywhere.

Ask yourself: 'Whose internal map am I following? Where did I stop trusting myself?'

Self-help: This is not failure; it's a turning point. Sit with the discomfort. Let quiet reveal what noise concealed. Getting lost is often how the soul recalibrates. You are not broken – you're simply rerouting. Be patient and trust that when the time is right you will find your right direction again.

48. Marriage or relationship problems

Dreams about divorce or relationship struggles aren't always about your partner. They often reflect a deeper emotional disconnect within yourself or a fear that your true feelings are being ignored or unseen in the relationship.

Ask yourself: 'What inner conflict am I avoiding? When did genuine connection start feeling like I'm just going through the motions?'

Self-help: It might be time to pour love back into yourself or to face where your relationship needs honest care, not just maintenance. These troubling dreams are invitations to reconnect first with yourself, then with each other.

49. Medical emergency or operation gone wrong

Medical-crisis dreams scream of broken trust in your body, others or the systems meant to help you. The healers may hurt or the fix makes things worse.

Ask yourself: 'What part of me feels wounded and who am I trusting to heal it? Am I being too trusting?'

Self-help: Slow down. Stop trying to be okay before you're ready. Ask for support but don't blindly trust or follow. Make your own mind up. Turn inward. Your body, your intuition . . . at the end of the day, they know what true healing looks and feels like.

50. Monsters

Monsters in dreams symbolize emotions you may have exiled – anger, grief, fear or shame made grotesque by neglect. The more you avoid them, the louder they roar.

Ask yourself: 'What emotion have I buried so deep it now feels monstrous? What part of me feels ugly?'

Self-help: Face it. Not with violence but with fascination and then compassion. Let the monster speak. These nightmares don't demand slaying they demand listening. Often, the thing you fear most holds the part of you that most needs love.

51. Murder or killing

Nightmares about murder or killing point to aspects of yourself that are being denied expression or an unwanted sudden change or something that feels forced upon you in waking life.

Ask yourself: 'What am I trying to end? What in your waking life do you feel is taking your decision to choose for yourself away?'

Self-help: Stop fearing the death of what no longer fits. Mourn, yes, but also make space. This nightmare marks a rebirth disguised as violent horror. What you kill in dreams may be what you no longer need to hold onto for survival.

52. Naked and humiliated

To stand naked and exposed in front of others in a dream is a primal nightmare. You're stripped of protection, dignity and safety and seen in all the ways you fear being judged or rejected.

Ask yourself: 'Why am I terrified of being myself? What or who is making me feel vulnerable or exposed?'

Self-help: These dreams don't mock you; they challenge you to own your truth. Shame feeds on silence. Practise small acts of authenticity and let vulnerability become your strength. The fear of exposure fades when you stop hiding and when you realize that most people are thinking about themselves, not about you.

53. Needles

Needle and injection nightmares pierce through emotional armour. Whether injecting pain or extracting something sacred, they symbolize your fear of betrayal, or emotional invasion.

Ask yourself: 'Where do I feel exposed? Do I feel punctured by someone's words, actions or expectations?'

Self-help: Don't dismiss the sting of this dream. Protect yourself with boundaries and care. These dreams are warnings – your inner self is aching for greater protection, healing and release.

54. Nuclear explosion

A nuclear blast in your dream symbolizes emotional obliteration – intense rage, grief or despair that has been buried for too long now threatens to erupt and cause total collapse. It's a critical tipping point: make or break.

Ask yourself: 'What emotional detonation am I postponing? What part of my waking life is on the verge of becoming unsustainable or breaking down completely?'

Self-help: Don't wait for a meltdown to force change. Take proactive steps towards healing and resolution. Speak the unspeakable if that's what it takes to reclaim your inner stability.

55. Obstruction or blockage

Nightmares of being blocked in some way – doors that won't open, elevators that stall – reflect internal paralysis. You're stuck – not because you're weak but because something vital inside is being ignored and you can't move on until it is addressed.

Ask yourself: 'What am I unwilling to confront? Is my self-talk helping or harming me?'

Self-help: Don't force your way out. Instead, look at what's blocking you and take your time to process and understand it. Fear is often the false wall between you and your next step. See it clearly. Move through it with loving intention.

56. Office horrors

Dreams of being fired or collapsing under work pressure reveal a nightmare of identity burnout. You're becoming a machine for productivity, not a human with purpose.

Ask yourself: 'What part of me is being sacrificed at the altar of career success? Am I taking on too much?'

Self-help: Burnout is a slow death. Rest isn't optional, it's lifesaving. Reconnect with who you are beyond your role. These dreams don't shame you – they beg you to stop betraying yourself and remember that on their deathbed nobody wishes they had spent more time at the office.

57. Pain

To feel the sensation of real pain in a dream is no accident. It's your psyche screaming what you've tried to silence within yourself – grief, shame, envy, anger, loss, betrayal.

Ask yourself: 'What have I numbed that still bleeds beneath the surface? What am I repressing that needs expressing?'

Self-help: Let it hurt. This inner pain doesn't mean you're broken – it means your truth is knocking. Don't put plaster on it. Listen to it. Healing begins when you stop pretending that you're fine, practise self-care and ask for support if you need it.

58. Paralysis

Paralysis dreams are soul-freezes. You want to scream, run, fight but you can't. Something in waking life has totally robbed you of voice, choice or will. You feel ineffective and utterly helpless.

Ask yourself: 'Where have I procrastinated or gone silent to survive? What is stopping me from moving on?'

Self-help: Reclaim momentum in tiny ways. A grateful thought. An honest truth. A whisper of curiosity. Paralysis dreams are symbols of your life suspended, waiting for you to wake it back up.

Paralysis nightmare – Yara

Yara had recurring dreams of lying paralysed, unable to scream or move as danger crept closer. She often woke in fear.

In reality, she felt voiceless in her academic and social circles, paralysed by anxiety and fear of judgement.

The dream reflected her emotional state: frozen and unable to assert herself. With therapeutic guidance, Yara began practising small acts of self-expression and assertiveness.

She learned to speak up in low-pressure situations and set boundaries with people who intimidated her. As her confidence grew, the nightmares faded. Her dream signalled the need to reclaim her agency and she did.

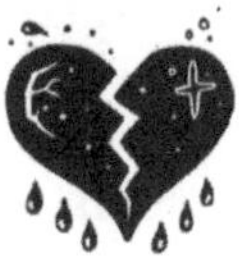

59. Partner cheating

Your partner betraying you in a dream is not a sign that they are actually betraying you – it's a symbol of your fear of abandonment, invisibility or emotional starvation.

Ask yourself: 'Where in my life do I feel unwanted, overlooked or insecure? Do I feel robbed of quality time with my partner or loved ones?'

Self-help: This isn't always about them – it's all about you. Your unmet needs. Your inner voice being ignored. Honour it. These nightmares don't prove betrayal; they reveal where you've been betraying your own heart.

60. People you dislike

When someone you despise or hate shows up in your dream, it's rarely about them – it's about the shadow they reflect. These figures often represent unhealed wounds, denied traits or boundaries you failed to enforce. They are signals from the unconscious, not villains.

Ask yourself: 'What part of me do I reject so deeply that it shows up wearing their face? What specifically about them is triggering such a strong reaction in me?'

Self-help: Don't suppress it, examine it. Reclaim what's yours. Release what isn't. This nightmare is a wakeup call, reminding you that the people who most provoke us in waking life often mirror our own unmet needs, disowned qualities or unresolved pain.

61. Phone malfunction

You're calling for help but the line is dead. Phone-failure dreams reflect poor communication and the feelings of panic, isolation or emotional abandonment this can trigger.

Ask yourself: 'Who am I desperate to reach? Why can't they hear me?'

Self-help: These dreams scream for emotional connection and better communication in your waking life, not just with others but with yourself. Speak even if your voice shakes. Listen even when it's uncomfortable. If no one answers, answer yourself. The silence is a mirror – face whatever it's showing you.

62. Plane crash

A plane crashing or veering off course in your dream symbolizes a collapse of control, ambition or self-belief. You may be aiming high – perhaps too high – and now fear the consequences of falling short or losing your way.

Ask yourself: 'What part of me is afraid of failure, exposure or being seen as not enough? What part of me needs to rise above the chaos and gain a clearer, higher perspective?'

Self-help: This dream is a call to stay calm under pressure. If the plane crashes, it's not the end – it's an invitation to rebuild with stronger wings. Ground yourself. Regain your sense of direction. This is not a symbol of destruction but a chance to fly again – this time guided by truth, not ego.

63. Pit or hole

You fall into a pit – dark, deep, inescapable. This haunting nightmare reveals buried emotions: isolation, depression or unresolved trauma. You may feel unseen, forgotten or emotionally trapped with no way out.

Ask yourself: 'What am I hiding from myself or the world? What pain am I carrying that makes me feel so alone or buried beneath it all?'

Self-help: Begin the climb – emotionally, spiritually, one small step at a time. Light doesn't return all at once, but the path out begins with a single breath, a single kind word to yourself. You are not truly alone, even if it feels that way. Reach out. Trust that healing starts with the decision to rise.

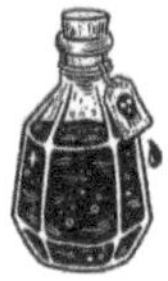

64. Poison

Dreams of poison whisper that something inside or around you may be polluting you without you realizing – until it is too late. Toxic people. Thoughts. Environments. Lies you've swallowed or allowed to grow.

Ask yourself: 'What am I consuming emotionally that's corroding my spirit? Are my thoughts and words healing or harmful?'

Self-help: Spit it out. Cleanse. Set boundaries. These nightmares are survival instincts, they're warning shots. Listen now, before there's real damage. You deserve to feel clean, whole and safe, and it starts with your next kind thought and word.

65. Police

When police or any law-enforcement officer is a threatening or menacing force in a dream, you're facing alarming inner or external judgement. Guilt, shame or fear of punishment looms large in your life.

Ask yourself: 'Who's policing my life? Is my inner critic stopping me in my tracks?'

Self-help: Dismantle fear-based authority inside your mind. You don't need permission from others to live your truth. These dreams demand that you reclaim your inner power, not through rebellion but through radical self-trust.

66. Possession

Being possessed by an invisible force or entity in a nightmare forces you to confront the parts of yourself you've disowned, like anger, grief or intuition, which may now demand your attention.

Ask yourself: 'What is controlling me that doesn't feel like my authentic self? What feelings have I buried that need to be reclaimed?'

Self-help: Begin the journey of reintegration by gently welcoming those disowned emotions back into your awareness. Healing comes from reclaiming your whole self with honesty and compassion.

67. Predator

The appearance of any kind of predator with evil intent in a nightmare often points to areas in your waking life where you feel exposed, threatened or overpowered, whether by external forces or internal forces like repressed anger, anxiety or shame. These figures represent both real and symbolic threats.

Ask yourself: 'Where in my life do I feel vulnerable or unprotected? What part of myself have I labelled as dangerous, unworthy or unacceptable?'

Self-help: Strengthen your emotional and mental boundaries. You are not helpless. Facing the predator – whether outside or within – is the first step towards reclaiming your safety, self-worth and personal power.

68. Public humiliation

A deep fear of rejection, exposure or failure is being symbolized here. These nightmares often surface when you're stepping into new roles or exposing your vulnerabilities and you fear judgement or being found out.

Ask yourself: 'What parts of me feel unworthy or shameful? Why do I feel I am not good enough?'

Self-help: Release the grip of perfectionism and shame. Your true power lies in your authenticity, not in flawlessness. Embrace your imperfections and let yourself be seen as you are. Light often enters through our cracks. You are enough.

Public-humiliation nightmare – Rosa

Rosa's nightmare involved standing before a crowd, suddenly forgetting everything she planned to say. The fear and shame were overwhelming. In waking life, she was under pressure at work and feared failure and judgement.

She realized the dream reflected perfectionism and deep fear of being 'exposed'. Using a combination of dreamwork and daily meditation, Rosa worked on self-compassion and reframed her relationship with failure.

She began rehearsing presentations in safe spaces and embracing imperfection. As her confidence grew, the nightmares disappeared. The dream taught her that being seen doesn't require perfection; it requires courage and authenticity.

69. Rape

Nightmares involving rape are deeply disturbing and often point to intense feelings of powerlessness, boundary violation or emotional invasion. For survivors of trauma, these dreams may echo painful memories and warrant professional support. Symbolically, they also highlight misuse of power when you feel used by others.

Ask yourself: 'Where in my life do I feel unsafe, unheard, used or violated? Am I being too passive?'

Self-help: Healing is possible. Seek compassionate support through therapy or grounding practices. Remember, this is not your fault. These dreams signal that a fierce inner courage is always trying to help you reclaim your voice and peace.

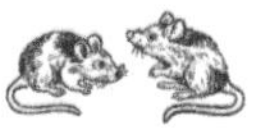

70. Rats or mice

Rats and mice in dreams symbolize anxieties or problems that undermine your sense of safety and peace. Guilt, betrayal or mental clutter you've tried to ignore but keep nibbling away at your wellbeing. Though tiny, they are persistent and adaptive survivors.

Ask yourself: 'What small issues or situations am I tolerating that wear me down? What emotional or physical clutter needs clearing?'

Self-help: Face your problems calmly, without panic. Begin by cleaning your inner and outer spaces. Addressing these small irritations can restore mental clarity and emotional calm, helping you feel grounded again.

71. Rejection

Dreams of rejection echo childhood wounds about belonging and acceptance. They reveal where you still allow others' opinions to define your self-worth, leading to self-denial and isolation. These nightmares ask you to examine how much you reject of yourself to gain approval.

Ask yourself: 'In what ways am I denying myself to be accepted? What would radical self-acceptance look like in my life?'

Self-help: Rejection themes in dreams can be a painful form of redirection. Embrace your wholeness and stop seeking permission to belong. True belonging begins when you accept yourself fully, without conditions. Do one thing each day that scares you. The path to success is paved with rejection because failure teaches us what does not work so we can course correct. Never be afraid to fail.

72. Robots

Robot dreams highlight emotional numbness or feeling trapped in rigid routines, acting on autopilot rather than engaging with life. These dreams reflect a loss of spontaneity, creativity and connection to your authentic feelings, often due to burnout or excessive pressure to perform.

Ask yourself: 'When have I become mechanical or disconnected? Am I going through the motions?'

Self-help: Break free from the programmed script.

Reclaim your humanity by embracing imperfection and creativity. Spend more time in nature. Listen to music that gives you goosebumps. Allow yourself to feel deeply and reconnect with your passions and find ways to tap into your intuition.

73. Running but not moving

Dreams of running, walking or climbing but somehow remaining in place express frustration and exhaustion, like a hamster wheel of effort that leads nowhere. You are expending energy on goals or relationships that no longer align with your true self, resulting in potential burnout unless changes are made.

Ask yourself: 'What am I chasing that no longer feels meaningful? Am I forcing a path that isn't right for me?'

Self-help: Step off the treadmill and pause. Rest and reflect on your direction. Sometimes, stepping back is the clearest way to regain strength and find a new path forward. Every day should be a new adventure, not a Groundhog Day.

74. Sand or quicksand

Dreams of sinking into sand or quicksand symbolize feeling trapped and unstable, as if every effort to move forward only pulls you deeper. These nightmares reflect situations – relationships, jobs or mental spirals – that drain your energy and sense of security.

Ask yourself: 'What weighs me down and holds me back? Am I fighting to fix what needs surrender instead?'

Self-help: Surrender doesn't mean defeat. It means softening your grip, letting go of the need to control what is beyond your control and asking for help. Find steadier ground through support and self-compassion. Sometimes stillness is the only way out.

75. Screaming or shouting

Dreams where you scream reflect intense emotions – anger, fear, grief or frustration – that are bottled up and not expressed in a healthy way in waking life. The loudness of your dream voice demands attention, signalling that you need to release these feelings instead of suppressing them.

Ask yourself: 'What emotions am I afraid to face or express? Who or what am I avoiding confronting?'

Self-help: Find safe ways to release your emotions, whether yelling into a pillow, journalling or creative expression. Letting your voice out is a vital step towards reclaiming your personal power.

76. Seizure

Seizure dreams indicate mental, emotional or physical overload and loss of control. They appear when you're stretched too thin, signalling burnout or breakdown. Your psyche uses these vivid images to warn you that your limits are being exceeded.

Ask yourself: 'Where am I ignoring signs of overwhelm? What part of me is shutting down?'

Self-help: Slow down and prioritize rest. Honour your body's needs and feed your mind with positive thoughts. Restoration is not optional – it's essential. Peace begins when you protect your own energy first.

77. Shadows

Shadowy figures in dreams symbolize repressed parts of yourself: anger, fear, pain or hidden power. They are not threats but aspects of you that are seeking acknowledgement. Ignoring them only gives them control, but facing them brings freedom and wholeness.

Ask yourself: 'What parts of myself have I denied or hidden? What truths do I fear seeing?'

Self-help: Engage in shadow work (see Chapter Three) through therapy, journalling or self-reflection. Embracing both light and dark within you allows true integration and growth.

78. Sharks

Shark dreams symbolize lurking emotional threats or anxieties circling you when you feel vulnerable. Sometimes the shark represents your own suppressed rage, fear or even ruthlessness waiting to surface.

Ask yourself: 'What fear is stalking me now? Is the threat real or imagined?'

Self-help: Trust your instincts and set clear boundaries. Sharks teach survival and resilience. You are not prey; you have the power to protect yourself and thrive.

79. Silent screaming or muteness

Dreams of screaming silently or being mute represent feeling voiceless and powerless to communicate effectively in waking life. These nightmares often connect to trauma, repression or fear of speaking your own truth.

Ask yourself: 'Where am I unable to express myself? Who or what has taught me to stay silent?'

Self-help: Start expressing yourself in small, safe ways through writing, trusted conversations or therapy. Your inner voice matters. Let it be heard, even if only in whispers and dream-journal entries at first.

Silent-screaming nightmare – Theo

Theo dreamed repeatedly of screaming in terror, but no sound came out. He woke feeling helpless and frustrated. In waking life, Theo struggled to express emotion, especially anger and sadness, fearing rejection.

The dream's silence mirrored his real-life emotional suppression. He asked, 'Where am I not speaking my truth?'

Through journalling, dreamwork and joining a support group, Theo slowly reclaimed his voice. He practised expressing feelings in safe environments and challenged the belief that vulnerability was weakness. As he opened up, the silent screams faded. His dream was not about fear – it was about finding the courage to be heard.

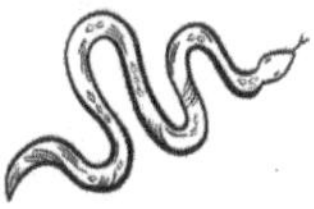

80. Snakes

Snake dreams evoke fear, temptation or what undermines and is not to be trusted, but they also suggest the potential for transformation and healing. They symbolize change and the shedding of old layers. Your emotional response reveals how ready you are to face growth and power.

Ask yourself: 'Where am I being undermined? What transformation am I resisting?'

Self-help: Avoid labelling the snake as purely negative. Embrace discomfort as a sign of awakening. Allow yourself to shed what no longer serves you and grow into new strengths.

81. Snowstorms

Dreams of snowstorms express a sense of isolation and confusion. The blinding snow buries familiar paths, reflecting feelings of being lost or frozen in place, cut off from warmth and support.

Ask yourself: 'Where am I emotionally overwhelmed or isolated? What or who am I avoiding?'

Self-help: Reconnect with sources of warmth – friends, nature, pets, comforting routines. Remember that snowstorms pass. Patience and connection can bring clarity and reveal new opportunities.

82. Spiders

Spider dreams often reflect feeling trapped – caught in webs of anxiety, manipulation, fear or relentless overthinking. But it's important to remember that spiders also symbolize patience, creativity, feminine power and strategic design. They are not only warnings – they are also teachers.

Ask yourself: 'Am I caught in a toxic situation or limiting pattern? Where in my life do I need to stop struggling and start creating with more intention and clarity?'

Self-help: Face your challenges with calm patience. Like a spider weaving its web, you can slowly and deliberately untangle what binds you. Rebuild your life with care, strategy and quiet strength, one strand at a time.

83. Stalked

Dreams of being stalked by known or unknown forces you cannot see often point to fears about what others think or to placing too much importance on external validation. These dreams may also reflect the internal pressure you put on yourself to meet unrealistic expectations or to appear perfect.

Ask yourself: 'Why do I prioritize what others think? Why do I feel I need to be perfect? Where did these beliefs come from?'

Self-help: Instead of constantly fleeing or avoiding

these feelings, begin to face them with curiosity. Talking to someone you trust, journalling your thoughts or gently exploring your emotions can help reduce the need to stay on high alert. Over time, this can create space for more self-compassion and less fear.

Stalking nightmare – Naomi

Naomi had nightmares of being followed through dark alleys by a silent stalker. She'd wake drained and anxious. In real life, she was avoiding a tough conversation with a close friend after a painful falling-out.

The stalker symbolized guilt and fear of confrontation – feelings she couldn't escape. Using her dream journal for inspiration, Naomi explored the emotions she was avoiding and asked: 'What am I afraid will happen if I speak my truth?'

She eventually reached out, initiating a heartfelt conversation. The act of facing her fear brought relief and the nightmares began to subside. The dream was her subconscious pushing her towards resolution, not avoidance.

84. Stranger danger

Menacing strangers in dreams symbolize anxiety about the unknown or unfamiliar aspects of yourself or your environment. These figures may also represent disowned qualities or the shadow you project outward.

Ask yourself: 'What feels threatening or foreign in my life? What parts of myself am I denying?'

Self-help: Set healthy boundaries but explore the unfamiliar with wonder rather than fear. Sometimes strangers carry important messages and can open you up to new perspectives you have not considered before. Protect yourself but be open to inner growth.

85. Struggle

Dreams of struggling physically – fighting, resisting, straining for your life – reflect internal conflicts or situations where effort yields little progress. This exhausting fight might be against yourself or external circumstances.

Ask yourself: 'Where am I fighting a losing battle? Does this struggle bring growth or only drain me?'

Self-help: Recognize what's beyond your control and what needs release. Sometimes the bravest act is choosing inner peace over battle. Rest, ask for help and nurture yourself instead of pushing harder.

86. Suffocating

Dreams of suffocation reveal emotional constriction and feeling trapped, silenced or overwhelmed. These nightmares arise when you cannot express your needs or feel stifled by toxic environments.

Ask yourself: 'Where do I feel restricted or silenced? Am I holding my breath to avoid conflict or please others?'

Self-help: Begin by breathing deeply, both physically and emotionally. Find safe ways to express your truth, even if you begin in small steps. You deserve freedom, space and to be both seen and heard.

87. Suicide

Dreams that feature suicide themes reflect overwhelming emotional pain – not necessarily a literal desire to die but a desperate urge for something to end. These nightmares may arise during periods of hopelessness, when you feel stuck, isolated or beyond help. They are cries from the psyche to release unbearable weight or escape a life situation that feels soul-crushing.

Ask yourself: 'What part of my life feels impossible to endure? What do I secretly wish I could end or walk away from?'

Self-help: You're not alone, even if the dream says otherwise. Do your dreamwork and your inner work. Speak to someone – a therapist, friend, hotline. Naming your pain opens a door to healing.

88. Teeth

Dreams that your teeth are shattering, crumbling or falling out are often linked to the fear of losing face or fears about your appearance. These dreams may arise when you feel you can't speak your truth or when you're under pressure to maintain an image that's cracking. There's a vulnerability here – your identity, confidence or control is under threat.

Ask yourself: 'Where do I feel voiceless or unable to hold it together? What part of me is not being assertive enough?'

Self-help: These dreams signal renewal. Let what's false or no longer in your best interests fall away. Speak up, even imperfectly. Strength often grows through what breaks. Assert yourself. You don't need to be toothless anymore.

89. Tornado

Tornado dreams represent sudden emotional upheaval and destruction spinning through your inner or outer world. You may be facing chaos, repressed emotions or an inevitable change on the horizon that terrifies you. The tornado doesn't wait for permission; it tears through what no longer serves.

Ask yourself: 'What area of life feels like it's spiralling out of control? What am I resisting that might actually be clearing space?'

Self-help: Ground yourself. Stay connected to simple routines, breathwork and supportive people. Once the storm passes, the landscape is changed forever – but it may be clearer and freer than before.

90. Torture

Torture dreams plunge you into scenes of extreme pain and violation. They may reflect inner torment – guilt, shame or trauma you carry silently. You could also feel punished in your waking life or trapped in a situation that continually violates your boundaries or spirit. They could be a sign you are at breaking point.

Ask yourself: 'Where do I feel emotionally or psychologically imprisoned? Am I being too harsh with myself?'

Self-help: Pain is real, but it doesn't need to define you. Acknowledge suffering and seek trauma-informed support if need be. You're not meant to live in agony – there is a life for you beyond the wound.

91. Toxic substances

Dreams involving chemicals, contamination or pollution reveal psychic damage. Serious emotional toxicity, perhaps negative people, unhealthy habits or damaging thoughts you've absorbed or allowed to gain momentum for too long. The body in the dream warns that something foreign and dangerous is inside you and you need to cleanse yourself of it.

Ask yourself: 'What am I taking in that poisons my inner peace? Who or what am I allowing to drain my energy?'

Self-help: Begin your psychic detox gently. Say no. Rest. Unfollow. Breathe cleaner mental air. Even a small act of clarity – drinking more water, stepping away, giving yourself more space – can signal to your system that it deserves care, not corrosion.

92. Tunnel

Tunnel dreams are claustrophobic but meaningful. You may feel confined, unsure when or if you'll reach the end. This darkness suggests a period of inner transformation – something old is dying but what's next isn't yet visible.

Ask yourself: 'What transition am I in right now? Am I mistaking passage for permanent imprisonment?'

Self-help: Trust the process. This tunnel may be guiding you, not trapping you. Light doesn't always appear immediately, but it does come. Stay with yourself, take small steps and let the dark be part of your becoming. Remember that at the end of every tunnel there is light.

93. Underground

You may feel emotionally deadened, overwhelmed or forgotten. These dreams can symbolize grief that has gone unspoken, trauma that has been pushed too far down or a desire to look deeper beneath the surface.

Ask yourself: 'What have I buried inside me to survive? Where do I feel unseen or erased?'

Self-help: Begin to unearth yourself slowly. Talk. Cry. Create. You are not meant to remain underground. What buries you now may one day nourish your emergence. Begin the climb back into air, light and life, and carry the lesson of this dream, which is that there is always deeper meaning to be discovered beneath the material.

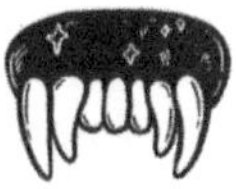

94. Vampire

Vampire dreams represent emotional or energetic depletion. Something or someone is feeding off your life force, leaving you tired, used or hollow. The vampire may also symbolize charm masking harm or your own seductive but draining habits.

Ask yourself: 'Who or what drains me while pretending to love me? Where in my life is my energy being drained more than it is replenished?'

Self-help: Protect your energy like blood. Set boundaries. Let rest and pleasure refill you. And don't fear your own inner hunger; just make sure you're feeding it from healthy, soul-affirming sources.

95. Violence

Violent dreams often highlight what you suppress: rage, fear, powerlessness. Whether you're the victim or the aggressor, violence represents parts of you in conflict, desperate to be heard. These dreams erupt when your emotional landscape has become very compressed.

Ask yourself: 'What anger have I denied? Where do I feel that I am invisible?'

Self-help: Find safe release and write furiously, punch pillows, scream into the wind. Violence in a dream doesn't make you violent. It means that something inside you needs out. Transform that inner fire into healing, not harm.

96. Vomiting or choking

Dreams of vomiting or choking reflect something inside you that can no longer be held or that does not nourish you. These are urgent symbols and whether it's a truth, emotion or memory, it needs to come out. Vomiting is expulsion. Choking is fear of saying what needs to be said.

Ask yourself: 'What's making me sick emotionally? What am I afraid to express or release?'

Self-help: You don't need to let it all out at once. Start the catharsis and the healing it will bring with a journal page, a single tear, a brisk walk, a talk with a supportive person. What you express won't destroy you; it will liberate you.

Vomiting and choking nightmare – Elias

Elias had recurring nightmares of uncontrollably vomiting and choking, unable to clear his throat. He woke in a panic. In waking life, Elias was overwhelmed, suppressing unresolved conflict at home.

The dream reflected his inability to express or release emotional pressure. Through therapy, he asked: 'What am I swallowing that I need to let go of?'

He began journalling, practising relaxation techniques and setting communication boundaries. Speaking openly with family also helped. As Elias processed his stress in healthier ways, the nightmares stopped. The dream taught him that holding things in was more painful than letting them out.

97. War

War dreams show up when your inner or outer world feels like a brutal battlefield. You may be locked in conflict – arguing, resisting, surviving something relentless. These nightmare scenarios reflect the toll of constant struggle and the urgent need for peace.

Ask yourself: 'What am I fighting for and is it worth the cost? Where could I start to lay down my weapons?'

Self-help: Prioritizing peace isn't weakness. Sometimes stepping away is the strongest thing you can do. Rest. Surrender control. Choose connection over conquest. Your inner world craves ceasefire right now.

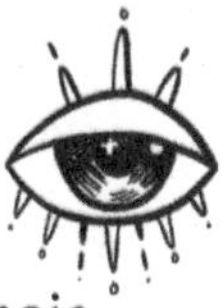

98. Watched by eyes

Dreams of eyes watching you suggest a sense of paranoia, shame or exposure. You may feel scrutinized by others or even by your own inner critic. There is no privacy here; every move is seen.

Ask yourself: 'Where do I feel judged or exposed? Whose gaze am I living under and is it my own or someone else's?'

Self-help: Reclaim your gaze. Turn inward, not with judgement but with curiosity and compassion. You don't have to perform or explain. Your worth isn't dependent on approval. Let yourself be free from imagined eyes watching you, as the only person you need to impress is you and the only eyes that you need to worship are your own.

99. You

Dreams where the grotesque or petrifying monster is you are disturbing for a reason – they reveal the part of yourself you've labelled as dangerous, shameful or unlovable. These nightmares ask you to stop running from your own shadow.

Ask yourself: 'What part of me do I fear the most? Is it possible that this darkness carries hidden wisdom, strength or truth I've been unwilling to face?'

Self-help: Your shadow isn't evil – it's unmet needs, suppressed pain and untapped power. Acknowledge it. Name it. Learn to work *with* it rather than against it. You are not the monster. You are the one becoming whole and learning to love even your sharpest edges.

100. Witches

Witches in dreams often stir fear of manipulation, curses or being controlled by unseen forces. But they also symbolize power, especially the intuitive, feminine or mystical power that has been denied, suppressed or misunderstood. This dream may reflect fear of another's influence or fear of your own gifts.

Ask yourself: 'Who or what in my life is scary and makes me feel powerless or manipulated? What part of my inner knowing or personal magic have I silenced or feared?'

Self-help: Engage with the witch archetype as a symbol of reclaimed power. Trust your intuition. Your power isn't dark – it's deep, ancient and wise. Learn to honour it, not fear it. Reclaim it with clarity and courage.

101. Zombies

Zombies represent numbness, burnout and emotional death. You're alive but not really living, maybe just going through the motions and feeling disconnected from joy, meaning and vitality. These dreams are a wakeup call from your soul.

Ask yourself: 'Where have I become lifeless? What parts of me are starving for passion or purpose?'

Self-help: Start small. One act of joy, one honest conversation, one deep breath. Reclaim your aliveness piece by piece. You're not the walking dead. This dream is calling you to wake up to the wonders of your precious life from the inside out, not the outside in.

Looking Up

Take a moment right now and if safe to do so, look up. Whether it's the ceiling above you, the sky beyond the window or just the open space overhead, give it your attention. Most of us spend our lives with our gaze turned downward towards the ground, our devices, our routines. We rarely look up. We rarely ask what else might be there.

But extreme dreamwork is about making a different choice. Not just with your eyes but with your whole way of being. It's about lifting your inner gaze. Choosing to rise above and use the perspective of your dreaming mind to always look higher. Choosing to see meaning where others see only mayhem.

In all 101 nightmares explored in this chapter, the perspective has been consistent: each dream, no matter how grotesque, terrifying or surreal, carries the potential to reveal something essential and potentially healing. This isn't about sugar-coating darkness. It's about refusing to waste it. Remember: when we approach nightmares with a willingness to understand, they shift from being sources of dread into sources of insight.

Every interpretation in this chapter leans into that possibility. Not because it's easy but because it's powerful. Seeing nightmares as messengers, rather than as threats, allows us to transform them into something constructive. This is the true alchemy of dreamwork: to turn discomfort into direction; to extract purpose from the very things that once overwhelmed us.

And here's the deeper truth: just like dreams, love and compassion are not passive experiences. They don't happen *to* us any more than dreams do. They too are choices we can make, even when it's most difficult to make them. But the struggle to redirect towards our inner light is worth it, because we open the door to a richer, more connected life.

So let this be your reminder: keep on looking up. Not just in your dreams but in your waking hours too. Why look at the ground when you can glimpse the stars? There is always something above you – something hopeful from the future waiting to be seen, something ready to guide you forward towards a higher, wiser and kinder version of yourself.

Conclusion

SWITCH ON YOUR NIGHTLIGHT

As we stand at the intersection of neuroscience and soul, we find ourselves revisiting ancient territory with new eyes. For thousands of years, cultures across the globe revered dreams as messages from beyond: gifts from the gods, ancestors or the deep well of the human soul. Before science attempted to label dreams as nothing but neurological static, we knew that night held something sacred. We treated dreams with reverence. Then, something shifted.

In a world that is increasingly rational and empirical, dreams were routinely dismissed and dream interpretation labelled 'woo-woo'. Nightmares were pathologized, medicated or ignored. We forgot that fear, when decoded with compassion, becomes insight. We forgot that the things that chase us behind our eyes and in our minds in the dark often lead us to the light. But we've had it backwards all along.

Those vivid dreams that shake us awake at 3am aren't neurological static – they're blessings. Those nightmares that terrify us? They may wear the costumes of wolves but underneath they're healers. Soul medicine wrapped in the shadow.

To face an extreme dream is to say: 'I'm strong enough to look at what hurts and isn't yet healed within me. I trust that even fear has wisdom and every pain has purpose.'

This is the power of extreme dreamwork. It doesn't just heal – it transforms. It shows that the parts of ourselves we try to exile are actually the parts that most need our love and understanding. Those brave enough to write down their dreams upon waking, to study the symbols, to face the fire, walk away not shattered but sovereign.

This book is all part of my ongoing mission to encourage everyone to reclaim their dreaming lives.

Dreams are not neurological leftovers. They are blueprints for becoming – soul maps for a more fulfilling waking life. Nightmares are not threats to peace; they are pathways to it. They arise when something deep within us demands to be seen, heard or healed. And while they may frighten us, they are also the dreams with the most transformative potential because growth lives in discomfort. Evolution doesn't arrive with roses, unless the roses have sharp thorns. True transformation often begins in our dreams, with broken teeth, with storms, with being chased by strange figures through the woods of the subconscious. These are extreme dreams – high-voltage transmissions from your deep, urging you to live deeper, feel more, be more. To honour them is to say, 'I'm ready.' Ready to face what you've avoided. Ready to grow. Ready to heal. Ready to shine.

In Neil Gaiman's *The Sandman,* the character Dream is not just a passive bystander to sleep. He is one of the Endless, an ancient, powerful force deeply invested in the consequences of the dreams humans weave for themselves at night. He is just, mysterious and protective of the sacred space of dreaming. Gaiman writes, 'Things need not have happened to be true. Tales and dreams are the shadow-truths that will endure when mere facts are dust.' Jung foreshadows this: 'We also live in our dreams we do not live only by day. Sometimes we accomplish our greatest deeds in dreams.'

Dreams are not echoes of waking life – they are calls to wake up to just how precious every moment of your waking life is. They speak in riddles and metaphors, yes, but the truth they hold is forever honest and real. And the more we listen, the more we learn, grow and heal. Too often, we run from 'bad' dreams. We avoid, repress, medicate. But, as you have discovered in this book, nightmares are urgent signals, transformative gifts. They arise when emotional wounds remain unhealed, traumas unprocessed, truths unsaid. These dreams are harbingers of change. The dreams that disturb us are often the dreams that can save us in every way.

Beautiful dreams of flying, dancing or reuniting with a lost love are blessings too. But it's the dark ones that do the deepest, most important work. The ones with fire, with teeth, with demons – that's where healing starts. Dark dreams help us identify limiting beliefs, process trauma, reclaim lost parts of ourselves, rewrite inherited stories and connect to our deepest wisdom. That makes dreamwork not just therapeutic but revolutionary. A form of inner activism. The more we explore extreme dreams, the more emotionally resilient, self-aware and self-loving we become.

Dreams Are Your Healing

If you take nothing else from this book, take this: your dreams – all of them, including the messy and extreme ones – *are* your healing. They are your intuition, your heart, speaking to you in symbols, questions and emotion. The more you honour them, the more you return to yourself and the inner peace that is your birthright.

Once you begin to truly listen to your dreams, your life begins to change. You become more awake at night and more alive by day.

If you've read or listened this far, you've done something brave. You've dared to walk through the darkest forests of your subconscious, to meet the wolves, the fires, the shadows within you. You've explored liminal states, danced at the threshold of life and death, listened to tales of trauma. You've learned that recurring nightmares don't haunt – they guide. That your inner child never wants to stop dreaming. That even beasts speak in metaphors and that you can learn to 'see' clearly in the dark. Most of all, you've come to know that every dream – most especially the ones you want to forget – carries a potential treasure for you to discover.

Closing Dreamwork Practices

As you continue your dreamwork journey, let these closing dreamwork rituals continue to support you and help you find your light in the darkest places.

The dream mantra

Repeat to yourself during the day: 'I look forward to meeting my dreams with love. I grow in my sleep. I dance and I heal in the dark.' This anchors your subconscious in trust and openness and you will carry that trust and openness into your dreams.

Dream altar

Create a small space with symbols of protection and creativity – crystals, candles, a quill pen, your dream journal. Let it be a nightly invitation to your inner world and a reminder that your dreamwork is sacred work.

A little nightlight

Keep a soft nightlight glowing. This comforts your present self as well as the inner child still wandering through all those old nightmares. Say: 'I am safe now. My dreams are here to help me, not hurt me.' This simple affirmation programmes your mind and heart to expect kindness, not chaos, from those dreams that come in the night.

The morning dream report

Upon waking, ask: 'What did my dreams want me to feel or know?' Don't rush. Let the insight rise gently.

Thank you for the dreams

Even the unsettling ones. After journalling your dream, place your hand on your heart and say: 'Thank you for showing me what I need to know.' Gratitude deepens the dialogue between your waking and dreaming selves.

See yourself down the dream road

Extreme dreams do not mean you are broken, deranged or haunted. They mean you are alive. That your soul still speaks, still aches, still hopes for great things for you. They are proof that something deeply honest within you is yearning to be understood, reclaimed, and transformed. There's a reason vivid dreams are such an effective reveal in films – through them, a glimpse of a character's inner truth is shown.

The greatest unexpected journeys you will ever take may not involve a map or a plane. They may begin in sleep. In symbols. In shadows. And perhaps the only thing standing between you and your next breakthrough is the dream you choose to stop running from.

So, tonight and every night, please welcome your dreams with open arms. Close your eyes not in fear but in awe. Keep your nightlight on. Somewhere on the other side of what is unknown, a wiser version of you is always waiting to embrace you. To dream is to dare. To face your extreme dreams is to evolve. In fact, drifting off to sleep might be the boldest adventure of all, since no one can ever touch or control your dreams.

So, keep on dreaming, my dear visionary friend. And from now on, may your dreams be not just sweet but dark, deep and extreme. As the extreme-dreaming pioneer Sigmund Freud once said: 'Dreams are often most profound when they seem the most crazy.'

Let your crazy dreams and the healing illumination they can bring into your night and your life forever shine on . . .

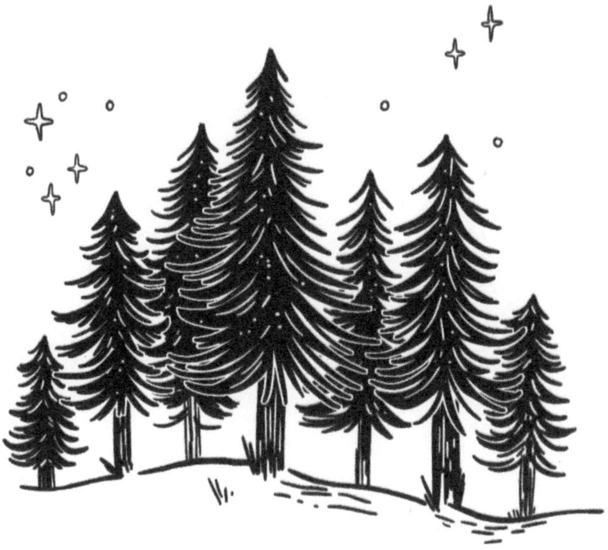

Acknowledgements

Thank you to my editor Louisa Johnson for her support and for being the visionary force behind this book of dreams; and to Rimsha Falak, Sarah Parry, Rosa Patel and Matilda Ngute at Octopus Publishing. Gratitude to my agent, Mark Gottlieb from Trident Media Group, for always being a dream to work with. And last but by no means least, special thanks to my readers and listeners for inspiring not just this book but all my books and my night visions too.

About the Author

Theresa Cheung is one of the world's leading dream decoders and spiritual authorities. Since graduating with a degree from King's College Cambridge, she has written numerous internationally bestselling titles, including two *Sunday Times* Top 10 bestsellers and *The Dream Dictionary from A to Z*. She has been named in Watkins' list of 100 Most Spiritually Influential Living People, is a go-to TV and media guest expert, a popular *White Shores* podcaster and host of UK Health Radio's *The Healing Power of Your Dreams*. You can email Theresa with dreamwork questions and stories via her website (www.theresacheung.com) or via her socials: @ thetheresacheung on Instagram, @thetheresacheungofficial on TikTok, or her Theresa Cheung author pages on Facebook and X. She aims to reply to everyone who reaches out as soon as she can but sometimes – especially when it's a full moon and dreams are said to be at their most extreme – response times may be longer.

'Is all that we see or seem but a dream within a dream?'

—Edgar Allan Poe

References

Citations – in order they appear in text

Brant Hasler and Anne Germain, 'Correlates and Treatments of Nightmares in Adults', *Sleep Medicine Clinics*, vol. 4,4 (2009), pp. 507–517. doi:10.1016/j.jsmc.2009.07.012.

Nicolas Deperrois et al., 'Learning Cortical Representations Through Perturbed and Adversarial Dreaming', *eLife*, 11 (2022), doi: 10.7554/eLife.76384.

Patrick Butlin et al., 'Consciousness in Artificial Intelligence: Insights from the Science of Consciousness', *arXiv*, 2308.08708 (2023) <https://arxiv.org/abs/2308.08708> [accessed 20 November 2025].

Phallab Ghosh, 'The People Who Think AI Might Become Conscious', *BBC News*, 26 May 2025 <https://www.bbc.co.uk/news/articles/c0k3700zljjo> [accessed 20 November 2025).

Jonas Mathes et al., 'Nightmare Distress is Related to Traumatic Childhood Experiences, Critical Life Events and Emotional Appraisal of a Dream Rather than to Its Content', *Journal of Sleep Research*, 32(3) (2023), pp. e13779, doi: 10.1111/jsr.13779.

Miti Sengupta and Rupam Banerjee, 'Creative Individuals Experience More Nightmares and Lucid Dreams: A Cognitive Inquiry', *International Journal of Dream Research*, 18(2) (2025), pp. 266–274, doi: 10.11588/ijodr.2025.2.111607.

Carlos Puentes-Mestril et al., 'How Rhythms of the Sleeping Brain Tune Memory and Synaptic Plasticity', *Sleep*, 42(7) (2019), zsz095, doi: 10.1093/sleep/zsz095.

Christian Cajochen et al., 'Evidence that the Lunar Cycle Influences Human Sleep', *Current Biology*, 23(15) (2013), pp. 1,485–8, doi: 10.1016/j.cub.2013.06.029.

Julia Mossbridge, 'Precognition at the Boundaries: An Empirical Review and Theoretical Discussion', *Journal of Anomalous*

Experience and Cognition, 3(1) (2023), pp. 5–41, doi: 10.31156/jaex.24216.

Clemens Speth and Jana Speth, 'A New Measure of Hallucinatory States and a Discussion of REM Sleep Dreaming as a Virtual Laboratory for the Rehearsal of Embodied Cognition', *Cognitive Science*, 42(1) (2018), pp. 311–333, doi: 10.1111/cogs.12491.

Patricia Tevington and Manolo Corichi, 'Many Americans Report Interacting with Dead Relatives in Dreams or Other Ways', Pew Research Center, 23 August 2023, <https://www.pewresearch.org/short-reads/2023/08/23/many-americans-report-interacting-with-dead-relatives-in-dreams-or-other-ways/> [accessed 20 November 2025].

Calvin E Cooper, 'Spontaneous Post-Death Experiences and the Cognition of Hope: An Examination of Bereavement and Recovery' (unpublished doctoral thesis, University of Northampton, 2017).

Garret Yount et al., 'Decreased Posttraumatic Stress Disorder Symptoms Following a Lucid Dream Healing Workshop', *Traumatology*, 30(4) (2024), pp. 550–558, doi: 10.1037/trm0000456.

Sandra Barreto, 'Near-Death Experiences: A Bibliometric and Systematic Review of Published Literature From 1977 to 2025', *OMEGA – Journal of Death and Dying*, 0(0) (2025), doi: 10.1177/00302228251363788.

Charlotte Martial et al., 'The Near-Death Experience Content (NDE-C) scale: Development and Psychometric Validation', *Consciousness and Cognition*, 86 (2020), pp. 1,053–8,100, doi: 10.1016/j.concog.2020.103049.

Marco Zanasi et al., 'Dreams and Age', *Perception and Motor Skills*, 100(3/2) (2005), pp. 925–38, doi: 10.2466/pms.100.3c.925-938.

Jonas Mathes and Michael Schredl, 'Gender Differences in Dream Content: Are They Related to Personality?', *International Journal of Dream Research*, 6(2) (2013), pp. 104–109, doi: 10.11588/ijodr.2013.2.10954.

Julia Mossbridge et al., 'Predictive Physiological Anticipation Preceding Seemingly Unpredictable Stimuli: A

Meta-Analysis', *Frontiers in Psychology*, 3 (2012), doi: 10.3389/fpsyg.2012.00390.

Jay Vera Summer, 'What Are Precognitive (Premonition) Dreams?', *Sleep Doctor*, 14 July 2025 <https://www.sleepfoundation.org/dreams/precognitive-dreams> [accessed 20 November 2025].

Julia Childs Heyl, 'When Dreams Merge with Your Waking Life – What to Know About Deja Reve', *Very Well Mind*, 20 November 2025 <https://www.verywellmind.com/deja-reve-8704831> [accessed 20 November 2025].

Jessica M Lust et al., 'Activation of Mirror Neuron Regions Is Altered in Developmental Coordination Disorder (DCD) – Neurophysiological Evidence Using an Action Observation Paradigm', *Frontiers in Human Neuroscience*, 13 (2019), doi: 10.3389/fnhum.2019.00232.

Jeffrey Long and Marjorie Woollacott, 'Long-term Transformational Effects of Near-Death Experiences', *Explore*, 20(5) (2024), doi: 10.1016/j.explore.2024.103030.

Index